An Inspirational One Year Record Keeping Journal

My Cancer Diary

Created by Robert John Keiber & friends

If found, please contact and return this book to:

_____ _____

Thank you.

Edited by

Ellen Thomas

Dedicated to my doctors and their staff:

Dr. Louis B. Harrison

Dr. Mark L. Urken

Beth Israel Medical Center

Institute for Head and Neck Cancer

Published by

The Tuxedo Group

Suite 2514

244 5th Avenue, NYC, 10001

212-252-2065

Introduction

If you are reading this book right now, it is most likely because either you have been diagnosed with cancer, or you are a person who cares very much about someone who has been diagnosed with cancer and you want to help. Either way you think this book will be of some benefit. You're right. It will be.

Let me say at the start that after my diagnosis I did feel like the Lone Ranger. There is a natural tendency to ask, "Of all the people in the world, why me?" If it is of any consolation, it is estimated that 40% of all Americans living today will be diagnosed with some form of cancer. That is approximately 92 million people. Today's cancer patient is not the Lone Ranger.

It can be a very lonely disease, none the less. Your friend gave you this book because he or she want to help, but doesn't know how. Don't close yourself off and don't chase away your friends, loved ones and partners. You will need them just to be there. My partner at the time moved in with me, and at many times I did get cranky, she was also frustrated by feeling that she could not do enough to help me. I told her that there was nothing practical she could do to cure me. My doctors and God were doing all that was necessary. But just being there was enough, because it can be a very lonely disease. My hospital roommate said to me once, "I'm lost, I just feel lost." I told him I knew exactly what he meant. I felt that way sometimes myself, even when surrounded by those who love you. I imagine that it is much harder to watch a loved one go through this challenge rather than to do it yourself. I was very grateful that I was diagnosed and not one of my loved ones. I'm not sure if I could handle that as well as my loved ones did. So go easy on them.

Even though studies make it clear that one's attitude and emotional state play key roles in the prevention of illnesses, these mental exercises should not be used to the exclusion of conventional medicine. Carefully choose the right team of doctors and follow their instructions. Be a curious student and a good patient. Relax, and try to be brave. There may be times when you feel you just can't be brave. You might find yourself depressed and even crying from time to time. I did, and I hadn't cried in years before that. Almost all of this will pass. Above all be patient. There's a reason why they call us patients. Use this book as a project to occupy your time. Use it as a record when you have to answer medical questions. Use this book as inspiration that will help you participate in your recovery. It is very important that you participate in your recovery with total intention of getting well. I hope the quotations and affirmations/meditations in this book will help you maintain your intention to recover. I had a participant in a workshop that I was giving ask, after hearing about my bouts with pneumonia and blood clots, "Weren't you afraid of dying?" I answered very honestly, "I never had any intention of dying. It just never occurred to me." Remember, nothing is as important to your recovery as your participation in it. Keep this record and make your journey a learning experience that you can pass on to those who follow.

"There is nothing the body suffers, from which the soul cannot profit by." - George Meredith.

How to Use This Diary

Unfortunately, even the best cancer doctors have too many patients to keep track of no matter how much they would like to. I used to ask my very good natured radiation doctor, Louis Harrison of Beth Israel in New York City, jokingly, "How's business?" He would reply with an exhausted look, "Too good." I remember waiting for hours to see my over-worked surgeon, Dr. Mark Urkin, as he almost ran from examination room to examination room trying to spend as much time as he could with each patient. I didn't like the wait, but I couldn't fault him. He certainly wasn't loafing while I waited. It was at this time I realized why they called us "patients." I took that time to read inspirational books, many of which are quoted in this journal. As the year progresses your patient file will get thicker and thicker with reports and records. Don't be afraid to ask for a copy of those reports.

One purpose of this diary is to keep you involved in your process by making notes of the vital information your doctor, his interns or his nurse practitioner will more than likely ask you upon each visit. As they rush from one patient to another they will want to know the **prescriptions** and **medications** you are on, the dosage, how long you have been on them, your last CAT/PET scan, chest x-ray, last visit and last surgery, etc. I kept an original journal like this one so that I could answer those questions quickly and accurately rather than have the doctor waste time looking through the voluminous file for the answers. Also under **things to do** note any questions you might want to ask the doctor or nurse which you might forget to ask during the visit.

Each day you open your diary you will be greeted with inspiration from the great positive thinkers of our time. Many of these thinkers are not only ancient sages, but medical doctors and researchers as well. Some are former cancer patients and survivors. Even if you think you are not "into being spiritual," try repeating these **meditations** 12 times or more each day. What can it hurt? You might think, "Oh, I'm just not that spiritual" or "I'm not really religious," or 'Wouldn't I be a hypocrite to turn to God now in my moment of distress." First of all, I don't believe God would hold it against you, and secondly, I'm not saying run out and get religion or join a church today. Let me just suggest that a little dose of God never hurt anyone. And if it works, then it works. If some other belief makes you feel good, go with it. The goal here is to feel good, at a time when feeling good is not so easy to do.

Remember to write down your brief **thoughts** for that day. You will think not only of your illness, but of life in general. Think of it as a personal guide for others to follow. Use it as a series of bench marks for your healing progress. As your health improves, and it will, use this journal as a reminder of how powerful your spirit and mind can be. You will change.

Doctor's phone number(s)

Dr.(GP)_____Dr._____

Dr._____Dr._____Nurse_____

Pharmacy_____Hospital_____Insurance_____

"Disease cannot live in a body that is in a healthy emotional state. See yourself living in a perfectly healthy body. Let the doctors look after the disease."

Bob Proctor

author, YOU WERE BORN RICH

"Let nothing disturb you. Let nothing frighten you. Everything passes away except God."

St. Teresa of Avila (1515-1582)

For a custom bookmark and gift card, personalized to the patient and signed by the author,

e-mail your name, address, and patients name to; *thetuxedogroup@yahoo.com*

For additional books by the author or information contact The Tuxedo Group;

thetuxedo group@ yahoo.com or call 212-252-2065

Other books available by the author at Amazon, Barnes and Noble, other online vendors and bookstores;

FEAR IS GOOD- *Overcoming stage fright.*

URBAN HYKOOL- *Haiku poetry exploring the Zen of the City.*

Good morning _____
Today your doctors and I
will be working on all your problems.
The only help we will need
from you is a positive attitude.
You work from the inside,
and we will work from the outside.
Have a good day.

God.

Questions You May Want to Ask Your Doctor in the Beginning.

1. Do you take my insurance?_____

2. What other tests will I need to confirm the diagnosis?_____

3. Will they be painful?_____

4. Where will they be done? (the office, the hospital, other)_____

5. If in the hospital, will I need to stay overnight, or be a day patient?_____

6. How soon will I know the results? Should I call you, or will you call me?_____

7. What treatments do you recommend? How long will treatments go on?_____

8. Will I need to be in a hospital for the treatments? How long?_____

9. Are there any clinical trials I should be aware of ?_____

10. How will my daily activities change during my treatments?_____

11. When will treatments start, what side effects should I expect and how long will they persist?_____

12. Who should I call if a side effect occurs and I am concerned?_____

13. Will I experience pain during these treatments?_____

14. What kind of pain management will I receive?_____

15. What medications will I need?_____

MY CANCER DIARY

"I think these difficult times have helped me to understand better than before how infinitely rich and beautiful life is in every way, and that so many things one goes around worrying about are of no importance whatever. "

**Isak Dinesen
author, OUT OF AFRICA**

Date:

Appointments:

Results/Reports:

Prescriptions:

Things to do:

Thoughts:

Meditation:

Thank you God, for this beautiful day

MY CANCER DIARY

"The decision to create is the decision to intend. To create healing, you can't have thoughts of illness and anticipate your falling victim to the disease. You can go within and hold an intention that says, "I want to feel good, I intend to feel good. I feel good. I refuse to allow any thoughts of disease or disorder in."

Dr. Wayne W. Dyer
author, THE POWER OF INTENTION

Date:

Appointments:

Results/Reports:

Prescriptions:

Things to do:

Thoughts:

Meditation:

 "Eternal Energy, awaken in me conscious will, conscious vitality, conscious health, conscious realization."

Paramahansa Yogananda

MY CANCER DIARY

"When people believe that life is meaningful and that they have a mission to accomplish they are strongly motivated to commit all their inner mind/body resources to help fight illness. That combination sometimes produces medical miracles."

Herbert Benson, MD
Harvard Medical School
co-author, TIMELESS HEALING

Date:

Appointments:

Results/Reports:

Prescriptions:

Things to do:

Thoughts:

Meditation:

"I have now transcended all patterns of illness, I'm free and healthy!

I am now full of radiant health and energy; I am energetic and full of vitality.

I am good to my body, and my body is good to me."

Shakti Gawain

author, CREATIVE VISULIZATION

MY CANCER DIARY

"We've learned that for every effect in our lives, there's a thought pattern that precedes and maintains it. Our consistent thinking patterns create our experiences. Therefore, by changing our thinking patterns, we can change our experiences."

Louise L. Hay
author, YOU CAN HEAL YOUR LIFE

Date:

Appointments:

Results/Reports:

Prescriptions:

Things to do:

Thoughts:

Meditation:

With a gentle hand I release regret. With acceptance I acknowledge lessons learned. With gratitude I give thanks for the richness of my experience. With a generous heart I share the treasures of my wisdom.

MY CANCER DIARY

"I'm a firm believer that hope and optimism are powerful forces in our lives."

**David B Agus, MD
author, A SORT GUIDE
TO A LONG LIFE.**

Date:

Appointments:

Results/Reports:

Prescriptions:

Things to do:

Thoughts:

Meditation:

Close your eyes and visualize white healing energy passing through the top of your head down through your body, passing into and through the distressed part of your body. Do not be alarmed if you feel a tingle, just continue and repeat for 5 minutes or more every day.

My mind is at peace.

MY CANCER DIARY

"There is nothing the body suffers which the soul may not profit by."

George Meredith (1828-1909)

Date:

Appointments:

Results/Reports:

Prescriptions:

Things to do:

Thoughts:

Meditation:

Visualize a place where you always felt safe and in a healing space, either from childhood, or even a favorite vacation spot at which you were happy, and at peace. Visit this place in your mind to comfort you when you are feeling badly.

MY CANCER DIARY

"Miracles do not happen in contradiction to nature, but only in contradiction to that which is known to us of nature."

St. Augustine (354-430 CE)

Date:

Appointments:

Results/Reports:

Prescriptions:

Things to do:

Thoughts:

Meditation:

I believe in miracles.

MY CANCER DIARY

"Guided imagery was one of the modalities on which, to my great surprise, I had found studies proving beyond a doubt that it could influence recovery rates for patients with cancer."

Candace B. Pert, PhD, Behavioral Neuroscientist
author, Molecules of Emotions

Date:

Appointments:

Results/Reports:

Prescriptions:

Things to do:

Thoughts:

Meditation:

My body is balanced, in perfect harmony with the universe. I give thanks for ever increasing health, beauty, and vitality. I am a radiant expression of God. My mind and my body now manifest divine perfection.

Shakti Gawain
author, CREATIVE VISUALIZATION

MY CANCER DIARY

"In my own practice, several cancer patients have recovered completely after being pronounced incurable and given only a few months to live. I didn't think they were miracles; I thought they were proof that the mind can go deep enough to change the very patterns that design the body. It can wipe out mistakes off the blue print and destroy any disease that disturbed the design."

Deepak Chopra, MD
author, QUANTUM HEALING

Date:

Appointments:

Results/Reports:

Prescriptions:

Things to do:

Thoughts:

Meditation:

(Quietly surrender yourself by creating positive thoughts that support your immune system. Love your body and send it loving thoughts that will penetrate you organs and your very cells, making them strong and powerful as they heal. See your body in perfect health every day. Move toward that image.)

I AM HEALTHY. I AM STRONG. I AM WELL

MY CANCER DIARY

"Certainly there are times in our lives when bad things happen, or when things don't turn out as we had hoped. But that's when we must make a decision to be happy in spite of our circumstances."

Joel Osteen, pastor
author, YOUR BEST LIFE NOW

Date:

Appointments:

Results/Reports:

Prescriptions:

Things to do:

Thoughts:

Meditation:

Today I will be happy. I am happy!

MY CANCER DIARY

"One of my patients, a 28 year old man, had experienced a complete remission from cancer after receiving a bone marrow transplant, but he hadn't slept for months. He was afraid he would never wake up. Guided imagery gave him a sense of peace that enabled him to release that fear. Soon he was able to get the restorative sleep he needed to stay well."

Mitchell L. Gaynor, MD
Weil Cornell Medical College
author, HEALING ESSENCE

Date:

Appointments:

Results/Reports:

Prescriptions:

Things to do:

Thoughts:

Meditation:

Nothing I see disturbs me. Nothing I see frightens me. I see a healthy, powerful person without fear.

MY CANCER DIARY

"At first I was scared and I didn't know how I was going to make it. I didn't think I was that strong. Then it struck me-even if only one per cent of people like me live, why couldn't I be in that one per cent?"

Eva Dupuy, survivor
Lung Cancer
HEALTHLINE MAGAZINE

Date:

Appointments:

Results/Reports:

Prescriptions:

Things to do:

Thoughts:

Meditation:

I am fearless and without limitations. I grow stronger each day.

MY CANCER DIARY

"Every detail of the belief system that we hold has consequences for better or for worse. It's for this reason that there is no such thing as an incurable or hopeless condition. Somewhere, at some time, somebody has recovered from it."

David R. Hawkins, MD, PhD
author, POWER VS. FORCE

Date:

Appointments:

Results/Reports:

Prescriptions:

Things to do:

Thoughts:

Meditation:

I feel great! I feel wonderful. My body is getting stronger and stronger every day!

MY CANCER DIARY

"Close relationships with friends and family members seem to have significant and highly beneficial effects on the immune system. Studies have linked happiness and positive emotions to longer survival among cancer patients."

Steven Locke, MD
Harvard Medical School
author, THE HEALER WITHIN

Date:

Appointments:

Results/Reports:

Prescriptions:

Things to do:

Thoughts:

Meditation:

(When you feel most alone, imagine your good friends gathered around you. They have their healing hands on your shoulder. They are whispering to you that you are very special and much loved.)

I hear you. I feel your healing warmth, and your gentle nurturing support.

MY CANCER DIARY

"One of the things I did to heal myself was to watch very funny movies. That's all we would do was laugh, laugh and laugh."

Cathy Goodman
Breast Cancer survivor

Date:

Appointments:

Results/Reports:

Prescriptions:

Things to do:

Thoughts:

Meditation:

Today I will laugh, and laugh, and laugh.

MY CANCER DIARY

We all come with a built in basic program of healing. It's called "self-healing." You get a wound, it grows back together. You get a bacterial infection; the immune system comes and takes care of those bacteria, and heals it up. The immune system is made to heal itself."

Ben Johnson, MD,
author, THE HEALING CODES

Date:

Appointments:

Results/Reports:

Prescriptions:

Things to do:

Thoughts:

Meditation:

I believe in the power of my mind to heal my body. I believe in the power of my spirit to heal my mind. I feel strong. I feel vital. Every day I am getting better and better.

MY CANCER DIARY

"Some of the most dramatic experiments putting hope and optimism to the test are those in which people unknowingly receive fake (placebo) treatments for real health problems and come out reporting they have improved just as much as those who got the real treatments"

David B. Agus, MD
author, ASHORT GUIDE TO
A LONG LIFE

Date:

Appointments:

Results/Reports:

Prescriptions:

Things to do:

Thoughts:

Meditation:

I know that everything in my life serves a purpose. I will only focus on the things that are positive

and that I need in my life. I will let go of all things I don't need in my life.

MY CANCER DIARY

"As long as the patient is convinced by his symptoms, he is caught up in a reality where "being sick" is the dominant input. The reason why meditation is so important in Ayurveda is because it leads the mind to a "free zone". Until you know that such a place exists, your disease will seem to be taking over completely."

Deepak Chopra
author, QUANTUM HEALING

Date:

Appointments:

Results/Reports:

Prescriptions:

Things to do:

Thoughts:

Meditation:

(Place your hands upon the affected part of your body. Close your eyes and visualize white healing energy passing through your head to your arms, to your warm hands. Concentrate the energy and the power of your positive thinking mind down to your warm, sensitive, healing hands.)

"The healing light of God surrounds me. The healing power of God flows through me. The healing love of God engulfs me. God is with me and all is well."

Shakti Gawain
author, CREATIVE VISULIZATION

MY CANCER DIARY

"Consider whence each thing is come, and of what it consists, and into what it changes, and what kind of thing it will be when it has changed, and that it will sustain no harm."

Marcus Aurelius, Emperor
of Rome. AD 121

Date:

Appointments:

Results/Reports:

Prescriptions:

Things to do:

Thoughts:

Meditation:

I now know that awareness is the very first step in healing. I will work toward becoming more aware each day.

MY CANCER DIARY

"In meditation the mind is held steady and not focused by grim determination, but by its own ability to enter into awareness once we stop distracting it. So how do we try to stop the stream of thinking? The answer is, you don't try. You decide to concentrate on your breathing."

David Fontana, PhD
author, MEDITATION

Date:

Appointments:

Results/Reports:

Prescriptions:

Things to do:

Thoughts:

Meditation:

I will rise above all negative thoughts and physical limitations. I will only focus on my healed strong body and mind.

MY CANCER DIARY

"People have been healing themselves and each other since the beginning. It's as if we've given some of our power away. Doctors contribute the expertise that is required for curing, but the healing happens with each other all the time. Healing is natural."

Rachel Naomi Remen, MD
author, THE HUMAN PATIENT

Date:

Appointments:

Results/Reports:

Prescriptions:

Things to do:

Thoughts:

Meditation:

Today is the future I create now.

MY CANCER DIARY

"Many studies and observations through the years have suggested the possible role of emotions in the etiology and course of cancer. There is ample evidence that psychological factors play some role in the genesis and the subsequent course of cancer once it has begun."

John E. Sarno, MD
author, THE MINDBODY PRESCRIPTION

Date:

Appointments:

Results/Reports:

Prescriptions:

Things to do:

Thoughts:

Meditation:

I blame no one for my disease, especially myself. I am one with the power that created me and with the help of this very same power I will transcend all patterns of illness.

MY CANCER DIARY

"At Stanford University, researchers showed Bizzaro comics to people while their brains were monitored by an MRI. They proved that humor stimulates the parts of the brain that use the "feel good chemical" dopamine. All the suggestions are that laughter is indeed good for you. So get those convulsions going and chuckle yourself to health."

William Weed, writer
READERS DIGEST

Date:

Appointments:

Results/Reports:

Prescriptions:

Things to do:

Thoughts:

Meditation:

As I consider the lives of Bob Hope, Milton Berle, George Burns, and Charlie Chaplin and how long they lived, I will start seeing the funny side of life and plan to live to a ripe old age.

MY CANCER DIARY

"Happier thoughts lead to essentially happier biochemistry, a happier healthier body. Negative thoughts and stress have been shown to seriously degrade the body and the functioning of the brain, because it's our thoughts and emotions that are continuously reassembling, reorganizing, recreating our body."

Dr. John Hagelin, PhD, quantum physicist

Date:

Appointments:

Results/Reports:

Prescriptions:

Things to do:

Thoughts:

Meditation:

I now release all angry negative feelings. I am willing to feel happy, healthy, and strong.

MY CANCER DIARY

"Our doubts and misperceptions, normal in any learning process, trigger the aches and pains we experience. Simply acknowledge this and then allowing our minds to change will in turn, change the way the body feels."

Karen Casey
author, THE COURSE

Date:

Appointments:

Results/Reports:

Prescriptions:

Things to do:

Thoughts:

Meditation:

I now choose to believe in my healing. I have power and authority over my body, my health, my mind, and my life.

MY CANCER DIARY

"On the other side of the equation are stories that reveal the power of a negative belief system, one of which was famously documented in 1974 when Sam Londe was diagnosed with terminal esophageal cancer. No one was surprised when he died a few weeks later despite treatment. But what did shock the medical community was the discovery upon autopsy that Sam didn't have esophageal cancer at all. Did thinking that he had terminal cancer cause his premature death?"

David B. Agus, MD
author, A SHORT GUIDE TO A LONG LIFE.

Date:

Appointments:

Results/Reports:

Prescriptions:

Things to do:

Thoughts:

Meditation:

(Picture yourself only in perfect health, with a golden healing light around the trouble body area(s). While touching the area with a warm hand repeat.)

"I am a radiant expression of God. My mind and my body now manifest divine perfection"

Shakti Gawain,
author, CREATIVE VISUALIZATION

33

MY CANCER DIARY

"We also begin to know that each of us is a part of all others, that no one walks alone, and that we are indeed at at home, and a part of the universe."

Lawrence LeShan
author, HOW TO MEDITATE

Date:

Appointments:

Results/Reports:

Prescriptions:

Things to do:

Thoughts:

Meditation:

I am not alone and I trust the power of the universe.

MY CANCER DIARY

"How we react depends upon the world we're reacting to. Who we become, as well as what we see, is determined by perception.-which can be said, simply to create the world."

David R. Hawkins, MD, PhD
author, POWER VS. FORCE

Date:

Appointments:

Results/Reports:

Prescriptions:

Things to do:

Thoughts:

Meditation:

The warm golden divine light within me is healing and creating miracles in my life here and now.

MY CANCER DIARY

If you believe that you are on the decline and will suffer and soon die, you may very well become a victim of a self-fulfilling prophecy. By the same token, if you believe that you can beat the odds, and enjoy a long life, you just might."

David B. Agus, MD
author, THE END OF ILLNESS

Date:

Appointments:

Results/Reports:

Prescriptions:

Things to do:

Thoughts:

Meditation:

I believe I will have a long healthy life

36

MY CANCER DIARY

"The body's ability to make sense of new information, to transform it, is health .If we are flexible, able to adapt to a changing environment, even a virus or damp air, fatigue or spring pollen, we can withstand a high level of stress."

Marilyn Ferguson
author, THE AQUARIAN CONSIRACY

Date:

Appointments:

Results/Reports:

Prescriptions:

Things to do:

Thoughts:

Meditation:

I am strong enough to survive.

MY CANCER DIARY

"The purpose of life is to live it, to taste experience to the utmost, to reach out eagerly and without fear for newer and richer experiences."

Eleanor Roosevelt

Date:

Appointments:

Results/Reports:

Prescriptions:

Things to do:

Thoughts:

Meditation:

My business is not to remake myself, but to make the absolute best of what God made."

Robert Browning

MY CANCER DIARY

"People grow old and die because they see other people grow old and die."

Shankara, Indian philosopher

Date:

Appointments:

Results/Reports:

Prescriptions:

Things to do:

Thoughts:

Meditation:

I feel young. I feel healthy. I feel strong.

MY CANCER DIARY

"Many cancer patients fall into the trap of getting depressed about getting depressed. Instead you must confront your depression and learn from it. No matter what, learn from the darkness-and accept that having cancer actually gives you a sense of freedom."

Bernie Siegel, MD
author, HOW TO LIVE BETWEEN OFFICE VISITS

Date:

Appointments:

Results/Reports:

Prescriptions:

Things to do:

Thoughts:

Meditation:

Today my real education begins. Today I will learn.

MY CANCER DIARY

"If you look under your depression, you will find anger. Look under your anger, and you will find sadness. And under your sadness is the root of it all, what's really been masquerading all the while - fear."

Carolyn Sterns
writer, PSYCHIC MASSEUSE

Date:

Appointments:

Results/Reports:

Prescriptions:

Things to do:

Thoughts:

Meditation:

I am afraid of nothing. I release all control to the Great Power of the Universe. I feel at peace with my body and my mind.

41

MY CANCER DIARY

"It is impossible for you to be angry and laugh at the same time. Anger and laughter are mutually exclusive and you have the power to choose either."

Wayne Dyer, PhD
author, YOUR ERRONEOUS ZONES

Date:

Appointments:

Results/Reports:

Prescriptions:

Things to do:

Thoughts:

Meditation:

I will heal myself with laughter.

MY CANCER DIARY

"Because magic seems so foreign to it, the rational part of our minds is generally quite fearful of the non-rational part....One is lead to believe that magical thinking is an act of healing, and that the most magical minds are therefore the healthiest."

Deepak Chopra, MD
author, UNCONDITIONAL LIFE

Date:

Appointments:

Results/Reports:

Prescriptions:

Things to do:

Thoughts:

Meditation:

I celebrate my body and rejoice in its health. I am strong, and glowing with power.

MY CANCER DIARY

"I rejoice in life for its own sake. Life is not a brief candle to me. It's a sort of splendid torch which I hold up for the moment and make it burn brightly as possible."

George Bernard Shaw

Date:

Appointments:

Results/Reports:

Prescriptions:

Things to do:

Thoughts:

Meditation:

I recognize my magnificent being. Like a glowing torch, I rise high above all my limitations.

MY CANCER DIARY

"That which we persist in doing becomes easier- not that the nature of the task changes, but our ability to do it has increased."

Ralph Waldo Emerson

Date:

Appointments:

Results/Reports:

Prescriptions:

Things to do:

Thoughts:

Meditation:

I will ask for what I want, again and again and again. I know I will receive what I need most.

MY CANCER DIARY

"We are not human beings having a spiritual experience. We are spiritual beings having a human experience."

Teillard de Chardin, philosopher

Date:

Appointments:

Results/Reports:

Prescriptions:

Things to do:

Thoughts:

Meditation:

My spirit lives in the perfect place at the perfect time. I will always be safe and secure.

MY CANCER DIARY

"Must we be vigilant every moment regarding the workings of our mind? Yes, but it's not as difficult as it may see to keep the mind in check. Fear is ever present when the mind wanders too far from God and love and the belief that we have purpose in this physical realm."

Karen Casey
author, THE COURSE

Date:

Appointments:

Results/Reports:

Prescriptions:

Things to do:

Thoughts:

Meditation:

I choose to feel no fear or pain today.

MY CANCER DIARY

"By the simple act of thinking vortexes are created, Invisible energies are are applied, and circumstances begin creeping to make real what was previously just imagined."

Mike Dooley
author, CHOOSE THEM WISELY

Date:

Appointments:

Results/Reports:

Prescriptions:

Things to do:

Thoughts:

Meditation:

I am becoming more and more aware each day. The more aware I become, the more I heal.

MY CANCER DIARY

"There is no stopping place in this life,-no, nor was there ever for any man no matter how far along his way he'd gone. This above all, then, be ready at all times for the gifts of God, and always for new ones."

Meister Eckhardt

Date:

Appointments:

Results/Reports:

Prescriptions:

Things to do:

Thoughts:

Meditation:

I am ready to accept the gifts of God.

MY CANCER DIARY

"In all good meditation, there is a therapeutic factor which is rarely mentioned. It is the careful paying attention to ourselves, to all ourselves, including those parts that we have characterized as the best and worst."

Lawrence LeShan
author, HOW TO MEDITATE

Date:

Appointments:

Results/Reports:

Prescriptions:

Things to do:

Thoughts:

Meditation:

I will explore myself and know myself.

MY CANCER DIARY

"The brain, which is composed of ten billion, billion working parts, has enough storage capacity to accept ten new facts every second. It has been conservatively estimated that the human brain can store an amount of information equivalent to one hundred trillion words, and that all of us use but a tiny fraction of this storage space."

Wayne Dyer, PhD
author, YOUR ERRONEOUS ZONES

Date:

Appointments:

Results/Reports:

Prescriptions:

Things to do:

Thoughts:

Meditation:

I control my brain. My brain does not control me.

MY CANCER DIARY

"Who you are is not somebody with cancer. Who you are is somebody-Somebody who matters."

Rachel Naomi Remen, MD
author, THE HUMAN PATIENT

Date:

Appointments:

Results/Reports:

Prescriptions:

Things to do:

Thoughts:

Meditation:

My mind and my body are always working toward health and happiness.

MY CANCER DIARY

"Today, mind/body interactions are accepted by many in the medical community. Recent studies show that stress-reducing techniques can cause measurable changes in the immune system."

**Medical Consensus Survey of 2000
leading cancer experts
PREVENTION MAGAZINE**

Date:

Appointments:

Results/Reports:

Prescriptions:

Things to do:

Thoughts:

Meditation:

I expect my life to be stress free, and filled with the joy of living.

MY CANCER DIARY

"All the evidence suggests that for most people chronic pain is a stress-related disorder, just like ulcers."

Dr. John Loeser, pain expert
University of Washington

Date:

Appointments:

Results/Reports:

Prescriptions:

Things to do:

Thoughts:

Meditation:

Today I will think of all the people I love, and that love me.

MY CANCER DIARY

"Maybe it's not really pain but a metaphor for anxiety and depression or spiritual suffering. We use pain for physical distress, and sometimes people don't make a distinction very well."

Elisabeth Rosenthal
author, "Chronic Pain", <u>THE NEW YORK TIMES</u>

Date:

Appointments:

Results/Reports:

Prescriptions:

Things to do:

Thoughts:

Meditation:

I always think positive. I expect good experiences. I deserve good experiences. Life brings me good experiences.

MY CANCER DIARY

"Optimism is like a muscle. If you exercise it on a regular basis, you can build it up. Before you go to bed think of three good things that happened that day."

Jeffrey Huffman, MD
contributor, MENS HEALTH MAGAZINE

Date

Appointments:

Results/Reports:

Prescriptions:

Things to do:

Thoughts:

Meditation:

I will monitor my minds work today. I will only remember good things.

MY CANCER DIARY

"The reason many psychological factors have been related to cancer is that they all induce internal rage. Work must be done on the source of the rage, not the rage itself. "

John E. Sarno, MD
author, THE MIND BODY PRESCIPTION

Date:

Appointments:

Results/Reports:

Prescriptions:

Things to do:

Thoughts:

Meditation:

The past has no power over me. I know the past is over and today I only live in the present.

MY CANCER DIARY

"We choose out joys and sorrows long before we experience them."

Kahlil Gibran, poet
author, THE PROPHET

Date:

Appointments:

Results/Reports:

Prescriptions:

Things to do:

Thoughts:

Meditation:

I choose a good life. I choose good health.

MY CANCER DIARY

"Most people don't recognize that the mind constantly chatters. And yet that chatter winds up being the force that that drives us much of the day, in terms of what we do, what we react to and what we feel. Meditation is a way of looking deeply into the chatter of the mind and body, and becoming more aware of patterns."

Jon Karat-Zinn, PhD
author, FULL CATASTROPHE LIVING

Date:

Appointments:

Results/Reports:

Prescriptions:

Things to do:

Thoughts:

Meditation:

I believe in perfect health. I believe in a healthy body. I believe in a healthy mind.

MY CANCER DIARY

"Cancer made me appreciate all that I have so much more. It taught me to enjoy every moment and to never, ever give up"

Ned Burns, survivor
Non-Hodgkin's Lymphoma
HEALTHLINE MAGAZINE

Date:

Appointments:

Results/Reports:

Prescriptions:

Things to do:

Thoughts:

Meditation:

I will rise above all negative thoughts and physical limitations. I will only focus on my healing, strong body.

MY CANCER DIARY

"What stands out about my experience are the relationships I have developed with my caregivers over the years. Let's face it, medicine is medicine, but if there's no relationship I don't think it's quite as effective."

Dorrie Bowden, survivor
Ovarian Cancer
HEALTHLINE MAGAZINE

Date:

Appointments:

Results/Reports:

Prescriptions:

Things to do:

Thoughts:

Meditation:

Today I will connect with someone special and treat him or her as a treasure.

MY CANCER DIARY

"At first I was scared and I didn't know how I was going to make it. I didn't think I was that strong. Then it struck me-even if only one per cent of people like me live, why couldn't I be in that one per cent?"

Eva Dupuy, survivor
Lung Cancer
HEALTHLINE MAGAZINE

Date:

Appointments:

Results/Reports:

Prescriptions:

Things to do:

Thoughts:

Meditation:

I will think big. There are unseen forces ready to help me in my healing

MY CANCER DIARY

"Perhaps the most powerful realization I had is that what is meant for me no one can take away from me. I believe I am meant to have goodness in my life, and I feel I have my whole life ahead of me to enjoy it."

Valerie Lee, survivor
Breast Cancer
HEALTHLINE MAGAZINE

Date:

Appointments:

Results/Reports:

Prescriptions:

Things to do:

Thoughts:

Meditation:

I gratefully receive loving care from others without fear or apologies.

MY CANCER DIARY

"No condition is anything more than a teaching tool. Whenever we learn something new, it changes ever so slightly how we view everything in our lives"

Karen Casey
author, THE COURSE

Date:

Appointments:

Results/Reports:

Prescriptions:

Things to do:

Thoughts:

Meditation:

My mind and my body are at peace today. I choose to feel great and be well.

MY CANCER DIARY

"My cancer taught me several important lessons. For one it taught me patience, because even though I decided I would be okay, I still had to go through all my treatments. It also taught me how to accept help from others. I had always been the person that helped everyone else; now it was their turn to be strong for me, and I think that helped all of us through the experience."

Valerie Lee, survivor
Breast Cancer
Healthline Magazine

Date:

Appointments:

Results/Reports:

Prescriptions:

Things to do:

Thoughts:

Meditation:

Today I will have patience with all things, but chiefly with myself.

MY CANCER DIARY

"Cancer has ultimately healed her sense of loneliness. I think what she means is that the process of being deeply wounded in this way has made her able to open herself to the love that is around her and that was always around her. This disease, in showing her vulnerability, has given her the gift of humanness. "

Rachel Naomi Remen, MD
author, THE HUMAN PATIENT

Date:

Appointments:

Results/Reports:

Prescriptions:

Things to do:

Thoughts:

Meditation:

My loved ones understand my needs. I have many people who love me.

66

MY CANCER DIARY

"I get up every morning and thank the person above that I am still alive. And I tell anyone, don't give up hope. It is truly remarkable, even with cancer, I've not missed a step in living my life."

Robert Hong, survivor
Stage 4 Colon Cancer
HEALTHLINE MAGAZINE

Date:

Appointments:

Results/Reports:

Prescriptions:

Things to do:

Thoughts:

Meditation:

Today I will only think of favors and gifts I have received in my life.

MY CANCER DIARY

"It's possible that if you live with fear, which many people do, day after day, month after month, the mechanisms that pump these natural "killer cells" [cancer fighting cells] into our bloodstream or increase their activity will get depleted over time. "

Margaret Kemmeny, PhD
Psychologist, University of Los Angeles

Date:

Appointments:

Results/Reports:

Prescriptions:

Things to do:

Thoughts:

Meditation:

I am not afraid. I will not live my days in fear.

MY CANCER DIARY

"Emotional fluctuations and emotional status directly influence the probability that the organism will get sick or be well."

**Candace Pert, PhD, Behavioral Neuroscientist
author, MOLECULES OF EMOTION**

Date:

Appointments:

Results/Reports:

Prescriptions:

Things to do:

Thoughts:

Meditation:

Today I visualize the challenge being over and my mind and body being peaceful.

MY CANCER DIARY

"If one person is saved one major operation by learning how to self-regulate using mind/body techniques, we've paid for most of the other patients in the clinic for the entire year."

Jon Kabat-Zinn, PhD
author, FULL CATASROPHE LIVING

Date:

Appointments:

Results/Reports:

Prescriptions:

Things to do:

Thoughts:

Meditation:

My body and my mind are in balance. I meet my challenge effortlessly with strength and flexibility.

MY CANCER DIARY

"Whatever your mountain is, you must do more than think about it, more than pray about it; you must speak to the obstacle. The Bible says, Let the weak say I'm strong. Let the oppressed say I am free. Let the sick say I'm healed."

Joel Osteen, pastor
author, YOUR BEST LIFE NOW

Date:

Appointments:

Results/Reports:

Prescriptions:

Things to do:

Thoughts:

Meditation:

I am strong. I am free. I am healed.

MY CANCER DIARY

"Coming to understand that situations appear as we project them will change how we feel. What we perceive as being external is created by us internally."

Karen Casey
author, THE COURSE

Date:

Appointments:

Results/Reports:

Prescriptions:

Things to do:

Thoughts:

Meditation:

I will select carefully what I project today. I will be blessed with a great day.

MY CANCER DIARY

"What stands out most about my experience are the relationships I have developed with my care givers over the years. Let's face it, medicine is medicine, but if there's no relationship I don't think it's quite as effective."

Dorrie Bowden, survivor
Ovarian Cancer
HEALTHLINE MAGAZINE

Date:

Appointments:

Results/Reports:

Prescriptions:

Things to do:

Thoughts:

Meditation:

I love, treasure and appreciate all my caregivers.

MY CANCER DIARY

"There is no question that your body and your mind tied together can help fight infection. Part of it is caused by lack of self-care, and I think part of it is a kind of turn off of the immune system."

Ron Anderson, MD
author, THE HEALING ENVIRONMENT

Date:

Appointments:

Results/Reports:

Prescriptions:

Things to do:

Thoughts:

Meditation:

I always treat my body with respect. I am good to my body and my body is good to me.

74

MY CANCER DIARY

"Miracles are mysterious and elusive. They have no characteristics. But the one element that is the same in all miracles is our change of thinking. Looking at it from this perspective suggests that we can create miracles at will. All we have to do is change our minds."

Karen Casey
author, THE COURSE

Date:

Appointments:

Results/Reports:

Prescriptions:

Things to do:

Thoughts:

Meditation:

I will overcome fear today. I will experience a miracle today.

MY CANCER DIARY

"I think a lot of the underlying physiology that explain the relationship between emotions and, for example the immune system, has to do with promoting the survival of the individual. . ."

Margaret Kemeny, PhD
Psychiatry Dept. UCLA

Date:

Appointments:

Results/Reports:

Prescriptions:

Things to do:

Thoughts:

Meditation:

I am not a victim. I am a victor.

MY CANCER DIARY

"Your words have enormous creative power. The moment you speak something out, you give birth to it. This is a spiritual principle, and it works whether what you are saying is good or bad, positive or negative."

Joel Osteen, pastor
author, YOUR BEST LIFE NOW

Date:

Appointments:

Results/Reports:

Prescriptions:

Things to do:

Thoughts:

Meditation:

I will only speak of the joy of living.

77

MY CANCER DIARY

"I truly believed in my heart, with my strong faith, that I was already healed. Each day I would say; Thank you for my healing. On and on I went, "Thank you for my healing. "I believe in my heart I was healed. I saw myself as if cancer was never in my body."

Cathy Goodman, cancer survivor
THE SECRET

Date:

Appointments:

Results/Reports:

Prescriptions:

Things to do:

Thoughts:

Meditation:

Thank you, God, for my strength and my healing.

MY CANCER DIARY

"It's common sense that what affects the mind or brain might have an impact on our health. You know we hear people say all the time, don't get yourself so stressed out that you become sick. They probably don't realize there is an actual biological basis for that."

David Fenton, MD, PhD
School of Medicine,
University of Rochester

Date:

Appointments:

Results/Reports:

Prescriptions:

Things to do:

Thoughts:

Meditation:

Today I will not stress over the little things. Today I will be grateful for the little things.

MY CANCER DIARY

"You pray in your distress and in your need. Would that you might also pray in the fullness of your joy and in your days of abundance."

Khalil Gibran, poet
author, THE PROPHET

Date:

Appointments:

Results/Reports:

Prescriptions:

Things to do:

Thoughts:

Meditation:

I thank you for my joy and abundance.

MY CANCER DIARY

"It is one of the most beautiful compensations in life that no man can try to help another without helping himself."

Ralph Waldo Emerson

Date:

Appointments:

Results/Reports:

Prescriptions:

Things to do:

Thoughts:

Meditation:

Today I will help myself by helping another in need.

MY CANCER DIARY

"Better one day of wise and thoughtful life than one hundred years of folly and thoughtlessness."
The DHAMMAPDA

Date:

Appointments:

Results/Reports:

Prescriptions:

Things to do:

Thoughts:

Meditation:

Today I will remove the word "victim" from my vocabulary and my thinking.

MY CANCER DIARY

"Dr. Constant Korotko, professor of physics at the St. Petersberg State Technical University in Russia, developed the Gas Discharge Visualization technique which could detect the electric soft colored light or "bio-field" surrounding a living organism. He concluded that every strong thought and emotion- whether love, hate, or anger- produced an extraordinary effect on the recipient."

Gary Schwartz, PhD
University of Arizona

Date

Appointments:

Results/Reports:

Prescriptions:

Things to do:

Thoughts:

Meditation:

I will monitor my mind's work today. What I think is all powerful.

MY CANCER DIARY

""We do not receive wisdom, we must discover it ourselves, after a journey through the wilderness which no one else can make for us, which no one else can spare us, for our wisdom is the point of view from which we come at least to regard the world."

Marcel Proust   (1871-1922)

Date:

Appointments:

Results/Reports:

Prescriptions:

Things to do:

Thoughts:

Meditation:

Each day I will become more patient and wiser.

84

MY CANCER DIARY

"Patient forbearance is the quality which enables us to prevent negative thoughts and emotions from taking hold of us. It safeguards our peace of mind in the face of adversity"

HH Dalai Lama

Date:

Appointments:

Results/Reports:

Prescriptions:

Things to do:

Thoughts:

Meditation:

I am healing more and more each day.

MY CANCER DIARY

"Deliverance depends on ourselves. There is no chance that others will deliver us, just as no one can stop the dreaming of a person asleep."

Longchenpa (1308-1363)

Date:

Appointments:

Results/Reports:

Prescriptions:

Things to do:

Thoughts:

Meditation:

My personal power will overcome this challenge.

MY CANCER DIARY

"For everyone who asks receives, and everyone who searches finds, and for everyone who knocks, the door will be open."

Mathew 7:7-8

Date:

Appointments:

Results/Reports:

Prescriptions:

Things to do:

Thoughts:

Meditation:

I want to be well.

MY CANCER DIARY

"No condition is anything more than a teaching tool. Whenever we learn something new, it changes ever so slightly how we view everything in our lives"

Karen Casey
author, THE COURSE

Date:

Appointments:

Results/Reports:

Prescriptions:

Things to do:

Thoughts:

Meditation:

My mind and my body are at peace today. I choose to feel great and be well today.

MY CANCER DIARY

"Have patience with all things, but chiefly have patience with yourself. Do not lose courage in considering your own imperfections, but instantly set about remedying them. Every day begins a task anew."

St. Francis De Sales (1567-1622)

Date:

Appointments:

Results/Reports:

Prescriptions:

Things to do:

Thoughts:

Meditation:

I am healing each day, little by little.

MY CANCER DIARY

"What lies behind us and what lies before us are tiny matters compared to what lies within us."

Oliver Wendell Holmes

Date:

Appointments:

Results/Reports:

Prescriptions:

Things to do:

Thoughts:

Meditation:

Today I will look within to find my strength.

90

MY CANCER DIARY

"A person's success or failure is not dependent on their circumstances. Many others are in the same situation. It is dependent on one's response to those circumstances."

Steven R. Covey
author, 7 HABITS OF HIGHLY EFFECTIVE PEOPLE

Date:

Appointments:

Results/Reports:

Prescriptions:

Things to do:

Thoughts:

Meditation:

Today I will find new ways of looking at my circumstances.

MY CANCER DIARY

"When you find positive meaning in every aspect of your life and start to realize that there is a greater force operating, you begin to develop the spirituality essential for true health."

Elliot Dacher, M. D.
author, WHOLE HEALING

Date:

Appointments:

Results/Reports:

Prescriptions:

Things to do:

Thoughts:

Meditation:

I recognize, respect and am in cooperation with a greater force without and within.

MY CANCER DIARY

"We don't have to make huge changes in our lives to begin feeling better. One act, one moment a time, will result in monumental changes before we know it. What can we do? We can smile always, instead of frowning."

Karen Casey
author, THE COURSE

Date:

Appointments:

Results/Reports:

Prescriptions:

Things to do:

Thoughts:

Meditation:

I will not succumb to pain or anger or despair today.

MY CANCER DIARY

"Our basic nature is to act, and not be acted upon. As well as enabling us to choose our response to a particular circumstance, this empowers us to create circumstances".

Steven R. Covey
author, 7 HABITS OF HIGHLY EFFECTIVE PEOPLE

Date:

Appointments:

Results/Reports:

Prescriptions:

Things to do:

Thoughts:

Meditation:

Today is a great day to be healthy.

94

MY CANCER DIARY

"Seventy five per cent of everything we think is negative, counterproductive and works against us. The brain simply believes what you tell it. You are what you think"

Shad Helmstetter, PhD

author, WHAT TO SAY WHEN YOU TALK TO YOURSELF

Date:

Appointments:

Results/Reports:

Prescriptions:

Things to do:

Thoughts:

Meditation:

I am in control of this situation. I will not think negative thoughts.

MY CANCER DIARY

"What we see or feel is only what's in the mind because thoughts are everything. We are responsible for our world, of course, and everything in it. Most of us aren't so eager to accept all that responsibility"

Karen Casey
author, THE COURSE

Date:

Appointments:

Results/Reports:

Prescriptions:

Things to do:

Thoughts:

Meditation:

Today I will only think the thoughts I want to think.

MY CANCER DIARY

"Each of us tends to think we see things as they are, that we are objective. But this is not the case. We see the world, not as it is, but as 'we are'-or as we are conditioned to see it."

Stephen R. Covey,

author, 7 HABITS OF HIGHLY EFFECTIVE PEOPLE

Date:

Appointments:

Results/Reports:

Prescriptions:

Things to do:

Thoughts:

Meditation:

I am worthy of health and happiness.

MY CANCER DIARY

"You might find yourself depressed and even crying from time to time. I did, and I hadn't cried in years before that. Almost all of this will pass. Above all be patient. There's a reason why they call us "patients."

Robert John Keiber, survivor

Date:

Appointments:

Results/Reports:

Prescriptions:

Things to do:

Thoughts:

Meditation:

Perfect health is the natural state of my body.

MY CANCER DIARY

"I know of no more encouraging fact than the unquestionable ability of man to elevate his life by conscious endeavor."

Henry David Thoreau

Date:

Appointments:

Results/Reports:

Prescriptions:

Things to do:

Thoughts:

Meditation:

I am enthusiastic about the adventures of today.

MY CANCER DIARY

"When the soul is in quietness it arises and leaves the body. And reaching the Supreme Spirit finds there its body of light. This is the land of infinite liberty, where, beyond mortal body, the spirit of man is free."

THE UPANISHADS

Date:

Appointments:

Results/Reports:

Prescriptions:

Things to do:

Thoughts:

Meditation:

I rise high above all my pain and worry to a place of peace and freedom.

MY CANCER DIARY

"When we turn our thoughts to peace, our ailments, whether physical or mental, or emotional, will recede. We are fortunate to have as much control as we have. It's awesome to contemplate how far-reaching our powers are."

Karen Casey
author, THE COURSE

Date:

Appointments:

Results/Reports:

Prescriptions:

Things to do:

Thoughts:

Meditation:

I am at peace in my body, if I am at peace in my mind.

MY CANCER DIARY

"Since the Lord is directing our steps, why try to understand everything that happens along the way?"
Proverbs 20:24

Date:

Appointments:

Results/Reports:

Prescriptions:

Things to do:

Thoughts:

Meditation:

My willingness to trust activates the power of God.

MY CANCER DIARY

"O mighty Ocean, I pray that the rivers of my desires, meandering through many deserts of difficulties, may merge at last in thee."

Paramahanda Yogananda

Date:

Appointments:

Results/Reports:

Prescriptions:

Things to do:

Thoughts:

Meditation:

I am asking for healing. I know it will take time. I have patience.

MY CANCER DIARY

"The appearance e of things change according to our emotions. And thus we see magic and beauty in them, while the magic and beauty are really in ourselves"

Kahlil Gibran, poet
author, THE PROPHET

Date:

Appointments:

Results/Reports:

Prescriptions:

Things to do:

Thoughts:

Meditation:

I will rise above my pain and see the magic and beauty around me.

MY CANCER DIARY

"In my eyes, the primary advantage of meditation lies in the fact that it is an entirely natural process- it allows the mind to discover its own subtlest layers without force, just as they discovered of calm quietness in normal life."

Deepak Chopra, MD
author, UNCONDITIONAL LIFE

Date:

Appointments:

Results/Reports:

Prescriptions:

Things to do:

Thoughts:

Meditation:

Today I will learn to be still.

MY CANCER DIARY

"To ease another's heartache is to forget one's own."

Abraham Lincoln

Date:

Appointments:

Results/Reports:

Prescriptions:

Things to do:

Thoughts:

Meditation:

Today I will look for opportunities of compassion.

MY CANCER DIARY

"If we had no winter, the spring would not be so pleasant: if we had no adversity, prosperity would not be so welcome."

Anne Bradstreet

Date:

Appointments:

Results/Reports:

Prescriptions:

Things to do:

Thoughts:

Meditation:

I will fight the good fight and win.

MY CANCER DIARY

"Every life situation teaches us something. Life situations always contain a message. And that message can be understood if we realize that life situations are providing us with the positive resources we need.

Chogyam Trungpa Rinpoche

Date:

Appointments:

Results/Reports:

Prescriptions:

Things to do:

Thoughts:

Meditation:

I will not accept pain, anger or fear today, but learn.

MY CANCER DIARY

"Begin with the end in mind is based on the principle that all things are created twice. There's a mental or first creation, and then a physical or second creation to all things,"

Steven R. Covey
author, 7 Habits of Highly Effective People

Date:

Appointments:

Results/Reports:

Prescriptions:

Things to do:

Thoughts:

Meditation:

What my mind can conceive my body can achieve.

MY CANCER DIARY

"Those who hope in the Lord will renew their strength. They will soar on wings like eagles; they will run and not grow weary, they will walk and not be faint."

Isaiah 40:31

Date:

Appointments:

Results/Reports:

Prescriptions:

Things to do:

Thoughts:

Meditation:

Today I will walk, tomorrow I will run, and the next day I will soar like an eagle.

MY CANCER DIARY

"Nothing happens to any man which he is not formed by nature to bear. The same things happen to another and either because he does not see that they have happened or because he would show a great spirit he is firm, and remains unharmed."

Marcus Aurelius, Emperor of Rome (AD 121-180)

Date:

Appointments:

Results/Reports:

Prescriptions:

Things to do:

Thoughts:

Meditation:

My mind and my body are strong today. I choose to feel strong today.

MY CANCER DIARY

"I have been driven many times to my knees by the overwhelming conviction that I had nowhere else to go. My own wisdom and that of all about me seemed insufficient."

Abraham Lincoln

Date:

Appointments:

Results/Reports:

Prescriptions:

Things to do:

Thoughts:

Meditation:

In time I will grow stronger.

MY CANCER DIARY

"By choosing your thoughts, and by selecting which emotional currents you will release and which you will reinforce, you determine the nature of the experiences of your life."

Gary Zukav
author, SOUL STORIES

Date:

Appointments:

Results/Reports:

Prescriptions:

Things to do:

Thoughts:

Meditation:

I choose healthy thoughts. I choose a healthy life.

MY CANCER DIARY

"There are no hopeless situations; there are only people who have grown hopeless about them."
Clare Boothe Luce

Date:

Appointments:

Results/Reports:

Prescriptions:

Things to do:

Thoughts:

Meditation:

I will no longer focus on pain or hopelessness.

MY CANCER DIARY

"To stop living in the past, to be healthy in mind, body and spirit, you must get up and move toward your future."

Joel Osteen. Pastor
author, YOUR BEST LIFE NOW

Date:

Appointments:

Results/Reports:

Prescriptions:

Things to do:

Thoughts:

Meditation:

I will use my pain as an advantage, and I will become a better person.

MY CANCER DIARY

"We must be very careful to control what we think. If you drive your car down an unfamiliar road and all you keep looking at is the detour barrier, instead of the path around the detour barrier, you will more than likely drive right into the detour barrier."

Robert John Keiber, survivor
Throat Cancer

Date:

Appointments:

Results/Reports:

Prescriptions:

Things to do:

Thoughts:

Meditation:

Today I will only see the path to healing.

MY CANCER DIARY

"Every time we create a positive shift in our perceptions of an event, we are contributing to the betterment of us all. How we see either heals or destroys."

Karen Casey
author, THE COURSE

Date:

Appointments:

Results/Reports:

Prescriptions:

Things to do:

Thoughts:

Meditation:

I see only good things today.

MY CANCER DIARY

"Eventually you will come to understand that love heals everything and love is all there is."

Gary Zukav
author, SOUL STORIES

Date:

Appointments:

Results/Reports:

Prescriptions:

Things to do:

Thoughts:

Meditation:

I am worthy of love, I am worthy of health and happiness.

MY CANCER DIARY

"One instant is eternity, eternity is now. When you see through this one instant, you see through the one who sees."

Wu-Men, Chinese Poet
Thirteenth-Century

Date:

Appointments:

Results/Reports:

Prescriptions:

Things to do:

Thoughts:

Meditation:

I look in the mirror I see a healthy strong person today.

MY CANCER DIARY

"The ancient guru told his disciples; All your suffering is rooted in one superstition. You believe that you live in the world, when in fact the world lives in you.-the mistake of the intellect"

Deepak Chopra, MD
author, UNCONDITIONAL LIFE

Date:

Appointments:

Results/Reports:

Prescriptions:

Things to do:

Thoughts:

Meditation:

I create the world I desire.

MY CANCER DIARY

"When the fear is taken away, people are empowered to deal with whatever they need to deal with and to seek and find meaning in the events of their life."

Rachel Naomi Remen, MD
author, THE HUMAN PATIENT

Date:

Appointments:

Results/Reports:

Prescriptions:

Things to do:

Thoughts:

Meditation:

Today I will create miracles.

MY CANCER DIARY

"Thinking health and wellbeing may not make a disease disappear, but the person's healed mind and attitude will guarantee a peaceful response to life."

Karen Casey
author, THE COURSE

Date:

Appointments:

Results/Reports:

Prescriptions:

Things to do:

Thoughts:

Meditation:

Today my mind will be at peace.

MY CANCER DIARY

"The real voyage of discovery consists not in seeking new landscapes, but in having new eyes."

Marcel Proust

Date:

Appointments:

Results/Reports:

Prescriptions:

Things to do:

Thoughts:

Meditation:

I am good to my body, and my body is good to me.

MY CANCER DIARY

"It doesn't take a hero to order men into battle. It takes a hero to be one of those men who go into battle."

Gen. Norman Schwarzkopf, survivor
Prostate Cancer

Date:

Appointments:

Results/Reports:

Prescriptions:

Things to do:

Thoughts:

Meditation:

I am a victor, not a victim.

124

MY CANCER DIARY

"Perhaps the most powerful realization I had is that what is meant for me no one can take away from me. I believe I am meant to have goodness in my life, and I feel I have my whole life ahead of me to enjoy it."

Valerie Lee, survivor
Breast Cancer
HEALTHLINE MAGAZINE

Date:

Appointments:

Results/Reports:

Prescriptions:

Things to do:

Thoughts:

Meditation:

I deserve a good life. I will have a good life.

MY CANCER DIARY

"The decision to create is the decision to intend. To create healing, you can't have thoughts of illness and anticipate your falling victim to the disease. You can go within and hold an intention that says, "I want to feel good, I intend to feel good. I feel good. I refuse to allow any thoughts of disease or disorder in."

Dr. Wayne W. Dyer, author
THE POWER OF INTENTION

Date:

Appointments:

Results/Reports:

Prescriptions:

Things to do:

Thoughts:

Meditation:

"Eternal Energy, awaken in me conscious will, conscious vitality, conscious health, conscious realization."

Paramahansa Yogananda

126

MY CANCER DIARY

"We move toward what we think about most. Unfortunately, it is just as easy to think about or move toward a vision of failure as it is to move toward a vision of success. Our thoughts control our behavior and our behavior validates our thoughts."

**Robert John Keiber, survivor
author, FEAR IS GOOD**

Date:

Appointments:

Results/Reports:

Prescriptions:

Things to do:

Thoughts:

Meditation:

I only have thoughts of health and success.

MY CANCER DIARY

"When people believe that life is meaningful and that they have a mission to accomplish they are strongly motivated to commit all their inner mind/body resources to help fight illness. That combination sometimes produces medical miracles."

Herbert Benson, MD
co-author, TIMELESS HEALING

Date:

Appointments:

Results/Reports:

Prescriptions:

Things to do:

Thoughts:

Meditation:

I have now transcended all patterns of illness, I'm free and healthy!

MY CANCER DIARY

"We've learned that for every effect in our lives, there's a thought pattern that precedes and maintains it. Our consistent thinking patterns create our experiences. Therefore, by changing our thinking patterns, we can change our experiences."

Louise L. Hay
author, YOU CAN HEAL YOUR LIFE

Date:

Appointments:

Results/Reports:

Prescriptions:

Things to do:

Thoughts:

Meditation:

With a gentle hand I release regret. With acceptance I acknowledge lessons learned. With gratitude I give thanks for the richness of my experience. With a generous heart I share the treasures of my wisdom.

MY CANCER DIARY

"Rather than give relief to the body, give relief to the mind. When the mind is at peace the body is not distressed."

Mumon (1900-1988)

Date:

Appointments:

Results/Reports:

Prescriptions:

Things to do:

Thoughts:

Meditation:

(Close your eyes and visualize white healing energy passing through the top of your head down through your body, passing into and through the distressed part of your body. Do not be alarmed if you feel a tingle, just continue and repeat for 5 minutes or more every day.)

I trust the process of life to heal me.

MY CANCER DIARY

"When left unexpressed and unresolved, emotions such as anger, hostility and feelings of loss and stress are dangerous to your health. So are feelings of helplessness… to insure your long term health, you need to take charge."

Elliot Dacher, MD
author, WHOLE HEALING

Date:

Appointments:

Results/Reports:

Prescriptions:

Things to do:

Thoughts:

Meditation:

Today I will take charge of my healing and my life.

MY CANCER DIARY

"There is nothing the body suffers which the soul may not profit by."

George Meredith (1828-1909)

Date:

Appointments:

Results/Reports:

Prescriptions:

Things to do:

Thoughts:

Meditation:

(Visualize a place where you always felt safe and in a healing space, either from childhood, or even a favorite vacation spot at which you were happy, and at peace. Visit this place in your mind to comfort you when you are feeling badly.)

I feel at ease, safe, and comfortable.

MY CANCER DIARY

"Miracles do not happen in contradiction to nature, but only in contradiction to that which is known to us of nature."

St. Augustine (354-430 ce)

Date:

Appointments:

Results/Reports:

Prescriptions:

Things to do:

Thoughts:

Meditation:

I believe in the existence of natural miracles.

MY CANCER DIARY

"Guided imagery was one of the modalities on which, to my great surprise, I had found studies proving beyond a doubt that it could influence recovery rates for patients with cancer."

Candace B. Pert, PhD, Behavioral Neuroscientist
author, MOLECULES OF EMOTION

Date:

Appointments:

Results/Reports:

Prescriptions:

Things to do:

Thoughts:

Meditation:

My body is balanced in perfect harmony with the universe. I give thanks for ever increasing health, beauty, and vitality. I am a radiant expression of God. My mind and my body now manifest divine perfection.

Shakti Gawain,
author, CREATIVE VISUALIZATION

MY CANCER DIARY

"No matter how successful we are, we all face challenges, struggles, and times when things don't go our way. When calamities occur, some people immediately think God must surely be punishing them. They don't understand that God has a divine purpose for every challenge that comes into our life. He doesn't send the problems, but sometimes he allows us to go through them."

Joel Osteen, pastor
author, YOUR BEST LIFE NOW

Date:

Appointments:

Results/Reports:

Prescriptions:

Things to do:

Thoughts:

Meditation:

I will search for meaning in my situation and I will grow healthy in spirit and body.

MY CANCER DIARY

"Reality is what we take to be true. What we take to be true is what we believe. What we believe is based on our perceptions. What we perceive depends on what we look for. What we look for depends upon what we think."

Gary Zukav
author, SOUL STORIES

Date:

Appointments:

Results/Reports:

Prescriptions:

Things to do:

Thoughts:

Meditation:

(Quietly surrender yourself by creating positive thoughts that support your immune system. Love your body and send it loving thoughts that will penetrate you organs and your very cells, making them strong and powerful as they heal. See your body in perfect health every day. Move toward that image.)

I see myself healthy. I see myself strong. I see myself well.

MY CANCER DIARY

"One of my patients, a 28 year old man, had experienced a complete remission from cancer after receiving a bone marrow transplant, but he hadn't slept for months. He was afraid he would never wake up. Guided imagery gave him a sense of peace that enabled him to release that fear. Soon he was able to get the restorative sleep he needed to stay well."

Mitchell L. Gaynor, MD
Weil Cornell Medical College
author, HEALING ESSENCE

Date:

Appointments:

Results/Reports:

Prescriptions:

Things to do:

Thoughts:

Meditation:

I am healthy. I am powerful. I am without fear.

MY CANCER DIARY

"Every detail of the belief system that we hold has consequences for better or for worse. It's for this reason that there is no such thing as an incurable or hopeless condition.-somewhere, at some time, somebody has recovered from it."

David R. Hawkins, MD, PhD
author, POWER VS. FORCE

Date:

Appointments:

Results/Reports:

Prescriptions:

Things to do:

Thoughts:

Meditation:

I feel great! I feel wonderful. My body is getting stronger and stronger every day!

MY CANCER DIARY

"Close relationships with friends and family members seem to have significant and highly beneficial effects on the immune system. Studies have linked happiness and positive emotions to longer survival among cancer patients."

Steven Locke, MD
Harvard Medical School
author, THE HEALER WITHIN

Date:

Appointments:

Results/Reports:

Prescriptions:

Things to do:

Thoughts:

Meditation:

(When you feel most alone, imagine your good friends gathered around you. They have their healing hands on your shoulder. They are whispering to you that you are very special and much loved.)

I feel your healing warmth, and I hear your gentle nurturing support.

MY CANCER DIARY

"Miracles can happen on a regular basis. We may often say, "I could sure use a miracle," How many times a day do we wish something different was happening? Miracles reside in the mind. What brings them about is our willingness to change how we perceive."

Karen Casey
author, THE COURSE

Date:

Appointments:

Results/Reports:

Prescriptions:

Things to do:

Thoughts:

Meditation:

How I think affects how I feel.

MY CANCER DIARY

"One of the things I did to heal myself was to watch very funny movies. That's all we would do was laugh, laugh and laugh. "

Cathy Goodman
Breast Cancer Survivor

Date:

Appointments:

Results/Reports:

Prescriptions:

Things to do:

Thoughts:

Meditation:

I truly believed in my heart, with my strong faith, that I am already healed.

MY CANCER DIARY

"Prayer is viewed as a kind of super-intention, a joint endeavor: you do the intending, and God carries it out. God puts the intention into action when you send out the intention."

Lynne McTaggart
author, THE INTENTION EXPERIMENT

Date:

Appointments:

Results/Reports:

Prescriptions:

Things to do:

Thoughts:

Meditation:

The light of God surrounds me. I intend to get well.

MY CANCER DIARY

We all come with a built in basic program of healing. It's called "self-healing". You get a wound, it grows back together. You get a bacterial infection; the immune system comes and takes care of those bacteria, and heals it up. The immune system is made to heal itself."

**Ben Johnson, MD
author, THE HEALING CODES**

Date:

Appointments:

Results/Reports:

Prescriptions:

Things to do:

Thoughts:

Meditation:

I believe in the power of my mind to heal my body. I believe in the power of my spirit to heal my mind.

MY CANCER DIARY

"What we think depends upon what we perceive. What we perceive determines what we believe. What we believe determines what we take to be true. What we take to be true is our reality."

Gary Zukav
author, SOUL STORIES

Date:

Appointments:

Results/Reports:

Prescriptions:

Things to do:

Thoughts:

Meditation:

I believe that everything in my life serves a purpose. I believe that a healthy body is my reality.

MY CANCER DIARY

"As long as the patient is convinced by his symptoms, he is caught up in a reality where "being sick" is the dominant input. The reason why meditation is so important in Ayurveda is because it leads the mind to a "free zone". Until you know that such a place exists, your disease will seem to be taking over completely."

Deepak Chopra, MD
author, Quantum Healing

Date:

Appointments:

Results/Reports:

Prescriptions:

Things to do:

Thoughts:

Meditation:

I feel the healing energy of the Universe surrounding me. I feel the healing power of God flow through me.

MY CANCER DIARY

"Consider whence each thing is come, and of what it consists, and into what it changes, and what kind of thing it will be when it has changed, and that it will sustain no harm."

Marcus Aurelius
Emperor of Rome. 121 CE

Date:

Appointments:

Results/Reports:

Prescriptions:

Things to do:

Thoughts:

Meditation:

I now know that awareness is the very first step in healing. I will work toward becoming being more aware each day.

MY CANCER DIARY

"In meditation the mind is held steady and not focused by grim determination, but by its own ability to enter into awareness once we stop distracting it. So how do we try to stop the stream of thinking? The answer is; you don't try. You decide to concentrate on your breathing."

David Fontana, Ph.D.
author, MEDITATION

Date:

Appointments:

Results/Reports:

Prescriptions:

Things to do:

Thoughts:

Meditation:

I will rise above all negative thoughts and physical limitations. I will only focus on my healed strong body and mind.

147

MY CANCER DIARY

"Many studies and observations through the years have suggested the possible role of emotions in the etiology and course of cancer. There is ample evidence that psychological factors play some role in the genesis and the subsequent course of cancer once it has begun."

John E. Sarno, MD
author, THE MINDBODY PRESCRIPTION

Date:

Appointments:

Results/Reports:

Prescriptions:

Things to do:

Thoughts:

Meditation:

I blame no one for my disease, especially myself. I am one with the power that created me and with the help of this very same power I will transcend all patterns of illness.

148

MY CANCER DIARY

"Smile. The act itself will trigger the release of pain-killing, brain happy endorphins and serotonin."

David Agus, MD
author, A SHORT GUIDE TO A
LONG LIFE

Date:

Appointments:

Results/Reports:

Prescriptions:

Things to do:

Thoughts:

Meditation:

As I consider the lives of Bob Hope, Milton Berle, George Burns, and Charlie Chaplin and how long they lived, I will start seeing the funny side of life and plan to live to a ripe old age. I will smile.

MY CANCER DIARY

"Happier thoughts lead to essentially happier biochemistry, a happier healthier body. Negative thoughts and stress have been shown to seriously degrade the body and the functioning of the brain, because it's our thoughts and emotions that are continuously reassembling, re-organizing, re-creating our body."

Dr.John Hagelin, PhD, Quantum Physicist

Date:

Appointments:

Results/Reports:

Prescriptions:

Things to do:

Thoughts:

Meditation:

I will release all angry negative feelings. I am willing to feel happy, healthy and strong.

MY CANCER DIARY

"Our doubts and misperceptions, normal in any learning process, trigger the aches and pains we experience. Simply acknowledge this and then allowing our minds to change will in turn, change the way the body feels."

Karen Casey
author, THE COURSE

Date:

Appointments:

Results/Reports:

Prescriptions:

Things to do:

Thoughts:

Meditation:

I now choose to believe in my healing. I have power and authority over my body, my health, my mind and my life.

MY CANCER DIARY

"While Westerners may consider subtle energy esoteric or New Age, it's been central to many healing traditions for millennia. Therapeutic touch (hands on –healing) has already been shown to accelerate wound healing and the immune system and to relieve pain. At New York's Presbyterian Hospital energy healers have been utilized during open-heart surgery."

Judith Orloff, MD
author, POSITIVE ENERGY

Date:

Appointments:

Results/Reports:

Prescriptions:

Things to do:

Thoughts:

Meditation:

(Picture yourself only in perfect health, with a golden healing light around the trouble body area(s). While touching the area with a warm hand(s).

My mind and my body now manifest divine perfection.

MY CANCER DIARY

"The most important treatment any healer can offer is hope for the health and wellbeing of those who suffer disease or trauma. Lack of faith in the power of Spirit to heal plays a deleterious role in the healing process."

**Wayne Dyer, PhD
author, THE POWER OF INTENTION**

Date:

Appointments:

Results/Reports:

Prescriptions:

Things to do:

Thoughts:

Meditation:

I trust the power of Spirit and the positive process of life to bring me to my excellent health.

MY CANCER DIARY

"When you interact with another, an illusion is part of the dynamic. The illusion allows each soul to perceive what it needs to understand in order to heal."

Gary Zukav
author, SOUL STORIES

Date:

Appointments:

Results/Reports:

Prescriptions:

Things to do:

Thoughts:

Meditation:

The warm golden light of my soul is healing my body.

MY CANCER DIARY

"Pessimists tend to have higher blood pressure and triglyceride levels than optimist have and their odds of a heart attack and early death are higher."

University of Pittsburgh study

Date:

Appointments:

Results/Reports:

Prescriptions:

Things to do:

Thoughts:

Meditation:

I am an optimist. I am optimistic about my health. I am optimistic about my life.

MY CANCER DIARY

"When people ask me if I was ever afraid of dying, I tell them it never crossed my mind. Even though I have been told I came close to death, I had absolutely no intention of dying."

**Robert John Keiber, cancer survivor
author, FEAR IS GOOD**

Date:

Appointments:

Results/Reports:

Prescriptions:

Things to do:

Thoughts:

Meditation:

I will get through this and be even better than before.

MY CANCER DIARY

"The purpose of life is to live it, to taste experience to the utmost, to reach out eagerly and without fear for newer and richer experience."

Eleanor Roosevelt

Date:

Appointments:

Results/Reports:

Prescriptions:

Things to do:

Thoughts:

Meditation:

Today I will make myself the absolute best of what God made.

MY CANCER DIARY

"Don't go to the neighborhood of despair: There is hope. Don't go in the direction of darkness: Sun exists."

Mellana Jalaluddin Rumi, poet
THE MATHNAWI

Date:

Appointments:

Results/Reports:

Prescriptions:

Things to do:

Thoughts:

Meditation:

I always move toward the light.

MY CANCER DIARY

"If you look under your depression, you will find anger. Look under your anger, and you will find sadness. And under your sadness is the root of it all, what's really masquerading all the while-fear."

Carolyn Sterns
writer, PSYCHIC MASSEUSE

Date:

Appointments:

Results/Reports:

Prescriptions:

Things to do:

Thoughts:

Meditation:

I am afraid of nothing. I release all control to the Great Power of the Universe. I feel at peace with my body and my mine.

MY CANCER DIARY

"There are many ways you can boost your positive outlook. Organized, deistic religions can achieve this, so can secular belief systems. All you need is a system that helps you to put even indescribable suffering into a wider context and tap into a higher awareness of yourself."

Deepak Chopra, MD
author, UNCONDITIONAL LIFE

Date:

Appointments:

Results/Reports:

Prescriptions:

Things to do:

Thoughts:

Meditation:

I seek a higher power to help me heal myself. I will seek a higher self to heal myself.

MY CANCER DIARY

"I rejoice in life for its own sake. Life is not a brief candle to me. It's a sort of splendid torch which I hold up for the moment and make it burn brightly as possible."

George Bernard Shaw

Date:

Appointments:

Results/Reports:

Prescriptions:

Things to do:

Thoughts:

Meditation:

I recognize my magnificent being. Like a glowing torch, I rise high above all my limitations.

MY CANCER DIARY

"That which we persist in doing becomes easier- not that the nature of the task has changed, but our ability to <u>do</u> has increased."

Ralph Waldo Emerson

Date:

Appointments:

Results/Reports:

Prescriptions:

Things to do:

Thoughts:

Meditation:

I will ask for what I want, again and again and again. I know I will receive what I need most.

MY CANCER DIARY

"We are not human beings having a spiritual experience. We are spiritual beings having a human experience."

Teillard de Chardin, Philosopher

Date:

Appointments:

Results/Reports:

Prescriptions:

Things to do:

Thoughts:

Meditation:

My spirit lives in the perfect place at the perfect time. I will always be safe and secure.

MY CANCER DIARY

"All bliss vanishes when the mind takes on suffering; all suffering vanishes when the mind takes on bliss. The reason this must be so is that our inner mirror, unlike one made of glass, actually becomes the image it reflects."

**Deepak Chopra, MD
author, UNCONDITIONAL LIFE**

Date:

Appointments:

Results/Reports:

Prescriptions:

Things to do:

Thoughts:

Meditation:

I see in my mirror today the image of a strong, healing person. I see the reflection of my healthy face, body and mind.

MY CANCER DIARY

"We come to understand that the situations appear as we project the changes of how we feel. What we perceive as being external is created by us internally."

Karen Casey
author, THE COURSE

Date:

Appointments:

Results/Reports:

Prescriptions:

Things to do:

Thoughts:

Meditation:

I will select carefully what I project today. I will be blessed with a great day.

MY CANCER DIARY

"To be ready for wholeness, first be fragmented. To be ready for fullness, first be empty. To be ready for renewal, first be worn out. To be ready for success, first fail."

Lao Tzu
author, The TAO TE CHING

Date:

Appointments:

Results/Reports:

Prescriptions:

Things to do:

Thoughts:

Meditation:

I am becoming more and more aware each day. The more aware I become, the more I heal.

I am healing more and more each day.

MY CANCER DIARY

"Acceptance without proof is the fundamental characteristic of Western religion. Rejection without proof is the fundamental characteristic of Western science."

Gary Zukav
author, SOUL STORIES

Date:

Appointments:

Results/Reports:

Prescriptions:

Things to do:

Thoughts:

Meditation:

My belief in my perfect health create my perfect health.

MY CANCER DIARY

"What if you slept? And what if in your sleep you dreamed you went to heaven and there plucked a strange and beautiful flower? And what if when you awoke, you had the flower in your hand?

Samuel Taylor Coleridge, (1772-1834)

Date:

Appointments:

Results/Reports:

Prescriptions:

Things to do:

Thoughts:

Meditation:

I choose to dream dreams of health and happiness. It is my divine right to do so.

MY CANCER DIARY

"Today, mind/body interactions are accepted by many in the medical community. Recent studies show that stress-reducing techniques can cause measurable changes in the immune system."

**Medical Consensus Survey of
200 leading cancer experts
PREVENTION MAGAZINE**

Date:

Appointments:

Results/Reports:

Prescriptions:

Things to do:

Thoughts:

Meditation:

**I expect my life to be stress free, and filled with the joy of living.
I am grateful for all the loving things that are given to me.**

MY CANCER DIARY

"All the evidence suggests that for the most people chronic pain is a stress related disorder, just like ulcers. "

Dr. John Loeser, pain expert
University of Washington

Date:

Appointments:

Results/Reports:

Prescriptions:

Things to do:

Thoughts:

Meditation:

Today I will think of all the people I love, and that love me.

MY CANCER DIARY

"Maybe it's not really pain but a metaphor for anxiety and depression or spiritual suffering. We use pain for physical distress, and sometimes people don't make a distinction very well"

Elisabeth Rosenthal, *writer*
"Chronic Pain", NEW YORK TIMES

Date:

Appointments:

Results/Reports:

Prescriptions:

Things to do:

Thoughts:

Meditation:

I always think positive. I expect good experiences. I deserve good experiences. Life brings me good experiences.

MY CANCER DIARY

"The reason many psychological factors have been related to cancer is that they all induce internal rage. Work must be done on the source of the rage, not the rage itself."

John E. Sarno, MD
author, THE MINDBODY PRESCRIPTION

Date:

Appointments:

Results/Reports:

Prescriptions:

Things to do:

Thoughts:

Meditation:

The past has no power over me. I know the past is over and today I only live in the present.

MY CANCER DIARY

"Round up all the people who are making you miserable and bring them to me. I will treat them as a counselor, and you will get better."

Wayne Dyer, PHD
author, POWER OF INTENTION

Date:

Appointments:

Results/Reports:

Prescriptions:

Things to do:

Thoughts:

Meditation:

I am independent, and not at the mercy of other peoples poor behavior. The road to love is forgiveness. I will forgive and travel on.

MY CANCER DIARY

"Most people don't recognize that the mind constantly chatters. And yet that chatter winds up being the force that that drives us much of the day, in terms of what we do, what we react to and what we feel. Meditation is a way of looking deeply into the chatter of the mind and body, and becoming more aware of patterns."

Jon Karat-Zinn, PhD,
author, FULL CATASTROPHE LIVING

Date:

Appointments:

Results/Reports:

Prescriptions:

Things to do:

Thoughts:

Meditation:

I believe in perfect health. I believe in a healthy body. I believe in a healthy mind.

MY CANCER DIARY

"Cancer made me appreciate all that I have so much more. It taught me to enjoy every moment and to never, ever give up"

Ned Burns, survivor
Non-Hodgkin's Lymphoma
HEALTHLINE Magazine

Date:

Appointments:

Results/Reports:

Prescriptions:

Things to do:

Thoughts:

Meditation:

I will dismiss all negative thoughts. I will only focus on my healed strong body and mind.

MY CANCER DIARY

"Perhaps the most powerful realization I had is that what is meant for me no one can take away from me. I believe I am meant to have goodness in my life, and I feel I have my whole life ahead of me to enjoy it."

Valerie Lee, survivor
Breast Cancer
HEALTHLINE MAGAZINE

Date:

Appointments:

Results/Reports:

Prescriptions:

Things to do:

Thoughts:

Meditation:

I trust that my life will be wonderful and filled with goodness and joy again.

MY CANCER DIARY

"In most lives insight has been accidental. We wait for it as primitive man awaited lightning for a fire. But making connections is our most crucial learning tool, the essence of human intelligence to forge links. To go beyond the given."

Marilyn Ferguson
author, THE AQUARIAN CONSPIRACY

Date:

Appointments:

Results/Reports:

Prescriptions:

Things to do:

Thoughts:

Meditation:

I will learn and I will heal.

MY CANCER DIARY

"I get up every morning and thank the person above that I am still alive. And I tell anyone, don't give up hope. It is truly remarkable, even with cancer; I've not missed a step in living my life."

Robert Hong, survivor
Stage 4 Colon Cancer
HEALTHLINE MAGAZINE

Date:

Appointments:

Results/Reports:

Prescriptions:

Things to do:

Thoughts:

Meditation:

I rise above all my limitations. Today I am inspired.

MY CANCER DIARY

"Make your positive imagery vivid with details. See them as real and replay the mental tapes over and over again. Use self-talk and positive imagery repeatedly, every day, to make the positive image easy to recall to the positive mind."

Robert John Keiber, survivor
author, FEAR IS GOOD

Date:

Appointments:

Results/Reports:

Prescriptions:

Things to do:

Thoughts:

Meditation:

I see the day of my recovery vividly every day.

MY CANCER DIARY

"It's possible that if you live with fear, which many people do, day after day, month after month, the mechanisms that pump these natural "killer cells" [cancer fighting cells] into our bloodstream or increase their activity they get depleted over time. "

Margaret Kemmeny, Ph.D.
Psychologist, University of Los Angeles

Date:

Appointments:

Results/Reports:

Prescriptions:

Things to do:

Thoughts:

Meditation:

Every experience I have benefits me.

180

MY CANCER DIARY

"Emotional fluctuations and emotional status directly influence the probability that the organism will get sick or be well."

Candace Pert, PhD, Behavioral Neuroscientist
author, MOLECULS OF EMOTION

Date:

Appointments:

Results/Reports:

Prescriptions:

Things to do:

Thoughts:

Meditation:

I am in charge of my life and my health.

181

MY CANCER DIARY

"If one person is saved one major operation by learning how to self-regulate using mind/body techniques, we've paid for most of the other patients in the clinic for the entire year."

Jon Kabat-Zinn, PhD
author, FULL CATASROPHE LIVING

Date:

Appointments:

Results/Reports:

Prescriptions:

Things to do:

Thoughts:

Meditation:

Today I take my life and my power back. Today I heal.

MY CANCER DIARY

"There is no question that your body and your mind tied together can help fight infection. Part of it is caused by lack of self-care, and I think part of it is a kind of turn off of the immune system."

Ron Anderson, MD
author; MEDICAL APERRTHEID

Date:

Appointments:

Results/Reports:

Prescriptions:

Things to do:

Thoughts:

Meditation:

I am patient, tolerant and I expect my life to be good.

MY CANCER DIARY

"Brains undergo a quite literal accelerated transformation. The transformative technologies offer us passage to creativity, healing choices.-The gift of insight for anyone willing to persist, experiment, explore."

Marilyn Ferguson
author, THE AQUARIAN CONSPIRACY

Date:

Appointments:

Results/Reports:

Prescriptions:

Things to do:

Thoughts:

Meditation:

Today I will transform my brain, and then my body, .

184

MY CANCER DIARY

"Coming to understand that the situations appear as we project them changes how we feel. What we perceive as being external is created by us internally."

Karen Casey
author, THE COURSE

Date:

Appointments:

Results/Reports:

Prescriptions:

Things to do:

Thoughts:

Meditation:

I will select carefully what I project today. I will be blessed with a great day.

MY CANCER DIARY

"Unto this darkness, which beyond light, we pray that we come, and through loss of sight and knowledge may we see and know that which transcends sight and knowledge, by the very fact of not seeing and knowing- for this is the real sight and knowledge"

DIONYSIUS (c. 500 CE)

Date:

Appointments:

Results/Reports:

Prescriptions:

Things to do:

Thoughts:

Meditation:

I will not accept pain, anger or fear today.

MY CANCER DIARY

"We shall not cease from exploration. And the end of all our exploring will be to arrive where we started, and know the place for the first time."

T.S. Eliot,
LITTLE GIDDING

Date:

Appointments:

Results/Reports:

Prescriptions:

Things to do:

Thoughts:

Meditation:

Today I will explore my body, my spirit, and my mind.

MY CANCER DIARY

"When we completely lose our way, we become one with loss. When we become one with loss, loss embraces us."

Lao Tzu
THE TAO TE CHING

Date:

Appointments:

Results/Reports:

Prescriptions:

Things to do:

Thoughts:

Meditation:

I am attentive and mindful to what is happening around me at all times.

MY CANCER DIARY

"Let it be like the rainbow, complete and free standing from the moment it appears, clear and bright with neither elation nor depression upsetting it."

Longchenpa, Tibetan Master (1308-1363)

Date:

Appointments:

Results/Reports:

Prescriptions:

Things to do:

Thoughts:

Meditation:

I will be firm and unshaken like a mountain, without fear.

MY CANCER DIARY

"To have his path made clear to him is the aspiration of every human being in our beclouded and tempestuous existence."

Joseph Conrad, (1857-1924)

Date:

Appointments:

Results/Reports:

Prescriptions:

Things to do:

Thoughts:

Meditation:

I see only health and goodness ahead of me. My life will be wonderful.

MY CANCER DIARY

"Life contains a lot of evils, as fragile as a bubble cast up by a wave and so how wonderful to wake up from sleep still breathing and say 'I am awake! There's still time!'"

ATISA, Tibet (982-1054)

Date:

Appointments:

Results/Reports:

Prescriptions:

Things to do:

Thoughts:

Meditation:

I create each day of my life as I want it to be.

MY CANCER DIARY

"The trial is a test of your faith, character and endurance. Don't give up. Don't quit. Don't whine and complain saying God, why is all this happening to me? Instead stand strong and fight the good fight of faith. God is giving you an opportunity for promotion. It is through the struggle that we find ourselves growing stronger."

Joel Osteen, pastor
author, YOUR BEST LIFE NOW

Date:

Appointments:

Results/Reports:

Prescriptions:

Things to do:

Thoughts:

Meditation:

I understand the challenge. I will meet it.

MY CANCER DIARY

"Smile! Smiling will boost your mood no matter what. The act itself will trigger the release of pain killing, brain-happy endorphins and serotonin. Besides, it's easier to smile; It takes seventeen muscles to smile and forty three to frown."

David B. Agus, MD
author, A SHORT GUIDE TO A LONG LIFE

Date:

Appointments:

Results/Reports:

Prescriptions:

Things to do:

Thoughts:

Meditation:

Today I will smile all day.

MY CANCER DIARY

"The spirit of life never dies. It is the infinite gateway to mysteries within mysteries."

Lao Tzu
TAO TE CHING

Date:

Appointments:

Results/Reports:

Prescriptions:

Things to do:

Thoughts:

Meditation:

My spirit life is strong. It brings me new understanding.

MY CANCER DIARY

"In every single cell of every human organism, the sum total of the whole life experience of every living organism since the beginning of time is preserved."

Sivik and Schoenfeld
microbiologists

Date:

Appointments:

Results/Reports:

Prescriptions:

Things to do:

Thoughts:

Meditation:

Today I will raise my soul so high, no discomfort or fear can reach it.

MY CANCER DIARY

"When the soul is in quietness it arises and leaves the body, and reaching the Supreme spirit finds then its body of light. This is the land of infinite liberty where, beyond its mortal body, the spirit of man is free."

THE UPANISHADS

Date:

Appointments:

Results/Reports:

Prescriptions:

Things to do:

Thoughts:

Meditation:

I am one with every power that created me.

MY CANCER DIARY

"It is for the sake of man, not God, that worship and prayers are required; not that God may be rendered more glorious, but that man may be made better."

Hugh Blair, England
(1718-1809)

Date:

Appointments:

Results/Reports:

Prescriptions:

Things to do:

Thoughts:

Meditation:

Divine peace and harmony surround me at all times.

MY CANCER DIARY

"Within the freedom to choose are those endowments that make us uniquely human. In addition to self-awareness, we have imagination-the ability to create in our minds beyond our present reality."

Steven R. Covey
author, **7 Habits of Highly Effective** *People*

Date:

Appointments:

Results/Reports:

Prescriptions:

Things to do:

Thoughts:

Meditation:

Everything I see and feel I create.

MY CANCER DIARY

"Do not chase after what is passed, do not worry over what is yet to come. The p is already thrown away, the future has not arrived. Simply grasp wholeheartedly what is here and now without wavering, without yielding. Look into it directly and realize it."

Buddha
THE MIDDLE WAY

Date:

Appointments:

Results/Reports:

Prescriptions:

Things to do:

Thoughts:

Meditation:

Every moment give me the opportunity to be growing and be well. I will stay in the moment.

MY CANCER DIARY

"Quiet minds cannot be perplexed or frightened, but go on in fortune or misfortune at their own private pace, like a clock in a thunderstorm."

Robert Louis Stevenson, Scotland (1850-1894)

Date:

Appointments:

Results/Reports:

Prescriptions:

Things to do:

Thoughts:

Meditation:

Today I will be calm and peaceful. Today I will become aware and insightful.

MY CANCER DIARY

"People ask me, when they told you that you had cancer did your whole life flash before you? The answer is no. I simply asked them, what are we going to do to cure it, and how soon could we start?"

Robert John Keiber, survivor
author, FEAR IS GOOD

Date:

Appointments:

Results/Reports:

Prescriptions:

Things to do:

Thoughts:

Meditation:

I intend to get well. The doctors and universe can take care of the detail.

MY CANCER DIARY

"What we imagine, we experience, and what we imagine affects us. It affects our immune system, and our strength, and our optimism. So we need to take control of our imagination and use it for our well-being."

Rachel Naomi Remen, MD
author, THE HUMAN PATIENT

Date:

Appointments:

Results/Reports:

Prescriptions:

Things to do:

Thoughts:

Meditation:

I create my own experiences. I create my health and strength.

MY CANCER DIARY

"If you call forth that which is in you, it will save you. If you do not call forth what is within you, it will destroy you."

St. Thomas

Date:

Appointments:

Results/Reports:

Prescriptions:

Things to do:

Thoughts:

Meditation:

I call forth my inner strength.

MY CANCER DIARY

"If we have the courage to listen, the willingness to feel, the ability to focus and the skill to remain present no matter what arises something amazing happens: our own authentic self emerges, moment to moment, in ways that are expected or surprising, convenient or challenging, but more importantly, and accurate reflection of who we really are in that moment."

Susan Piver
author, THE HARD QUESTIONS FOR
AN AUTHENTIC LIFE

Date:

Appointments:

Results/Reports:

Prescriptions:

Things to do:

Thoughts:

Meditation:

Today I will listen. Feel and focus to find out who I am.

MY CANCER DIARY

"Spirituality I take to be concerned with those qualities of the human spirit-such as love, compassion, patience, tolerance, forgiveness, contentment, a sense of responsibility, a sense of harmony-which bring happiness to both self and others."

The Dalai Lama,
author, ETHICS FOR THE NEW MILLENIUM

Date:

Appointments:

Results/Reports:

Prescriptions:

Things to do:

Thoughts:

Meditation:

Today I will begin to explore my spirituality.

MY CANCER DIARY

"Let part of thy soul which leads and governs be undisturbed by movements in the flesh whether of pleasure or of pain; let it not untie with them,"

Marcus Aurelius
Emperor Rome 121 CE

Date:

Appointments:

Results/Reports:

Prescriptions:

Things to do:

Thoughts:

Meditation:

My body does not control my soul.

MY CANCER DIARY

"An illness is a localized form of unease (as the term "dis-ease" implies), and it is not surprising to find that for many people, a much broader unease underlies it."

Deepak Chopra, MD
author, UNCONDITIONAL LIFE

Date:

Appointments:

Results/Reports:

Prescriptions:

Things to do:

Thoughts:

Meditation:

Today I release all thoughts and concerns which make me uneasy.

MY CANCER DIARY

"Our thoughts, our words, and our deeds are the threads of the net which we throw around ourselves."

Swami Vivekananda

Date:

Appointments:

Results/Reports:

Prescriptions:

Things to do:

Thoughts:

Meditation:

I will not trap myself with negative words and thoughts.

MY CANCER DIARY

"Through meditation you will learn to experience the field of pure silence and pure awareness. In that field of pure silence is the field of infinite correlation, the field of infinite organizing power, the ultimate ground of creation where everything is inseparably connected with everything else."

Deepak Chopra, MD
author, THE SEVEN SPIRITUAL
LAWS OF SUCESS

Date:

Appointments:

Results/Reports:

Prescriptions:

Things to do:

Thoughts:

Meditation:

Today I will start to meditate

MY CANCER DIARY

"The ability to feel pleasure is in itself a creative act. Think about what truly brings you delight. Deep pleasure, even joy, results from rousing your own creativity"

Susan Piver
author, HARD QUESTIONS FOR
AN AUTHENTIC LIFE

Date:

Appointments:

Results/Reports:

Prescriptions:

Things to do:

Thoughts:

Meditation:

Today I will create pleasure for myself and those around me.

MY CANCER DIARY

"The difference in power between a loving thought and a fearful thought is so enormous as to be beyond the capacity of the human imagination to easily comprehend. We can also see, however, that even a few loving thoughts during the course of the day more than counterbalance all our negative thoughts."

David R. Hawkins, MD, PhD
author, POWER VS. FORCE

Date:

Appointments:

Results/Reports:

Prescriptions:

Things to do:

Thoughts:

Meditation:

I will replace all my fearful thoughts with loving thoughts today.

MY CANCER DIARY

"There is nothing to worry about! Absolutely nothing. You can spend the rest of your life, begging right now, worrying about the future, and no amount of worry will change a thing. If you are planning, and the present-moment   activity will contribute to a more effective future, then this is not worry."

Wayne Dyer, PhD
author, YOUR ERRONEOUS ZONES

Date:

Appointments:

Results/Reports:

Prescriptions:

Things to do:

Thoughts:

Meditation:

Today I will plan for a healthy future, but not worry.

MY CANCER DIARY

"There is a growing body of evidence, much of it European, which suggests that emotional history is extremely important in things like the incidence of cancer."

**Candace Pert, PhD, Behavioral Neuroscientist
author, MOLECULES OF EMOTION**

Date:

Appointments:

Results/Reports:

Prescriptions:

Things to do:

Thoughts:

Meditation:

Today I will heal myself by letting go of all past grudges and forgiving others.

MY CANCER DIARY

"However, it was Dr. Diamond's demonstration that the body instantly went weak in response to unhealthy emotional attitudes or mental stresses that had the greatest clinical influences."

David R. Hawkins, MD, PhD
author, POWER VS. FORCE

Date:

Appointments:

Results/Reports:

Prescriptions:

Things to do:

Thoughts:

Meditation:

I am emotionally healthy and emotional strong.

MY CANCER DIARY

"I truly believed in my heart, with my strong faith, that I was already healed. Each day I would say," Thank you for my healing." On and on I went, "Thank you for my healing." I believe in my heart I was healed. I saw myself as if cancer was never in my body."

**Cathy Goodman, cancer survivor
contributor, THE SECRET**

Date:

Appointments:

Results/Reports:

Prescriptions:

Things to do:

Thoughts:

Meditation:

I will not accept pain, anger or fear today.

MY CANCER DIARY

"To have compassion for oneself and for all of mankind is instrumental-not only for recovery, but for any major advancement of consciousness.-as we go through the painful struggles of evolution. Only then do we become healers as well as healed, and only then to we hope to be cured of any malaise, physical or spiritual."

**David R. Hawkins, MD, PhD
author, POWER VS. FORCE**

Date:

Appointments:

Results/Reports:

Prescriptions:

Things to do:

Thoughts:

Meditation:

Today I will heal by concerning myself with the healing of others.

MY CANCER DIARY

"By taking responsibility for the consequences of his own perceptions, the observer can transcend the role of victim to an understanding that; nothing out there has power over you."

David R. Hawkins, MD, PhD
author, POWER VS. FORCE

Date:

Appointments:

Results/Reports:

Prescriptions:

Things to do:

Thoughts:

Meditation:

I am responsible for my healing.

MY CANCER DIARY

"It isn't life's events, but how one reacts to them and the attitude that one has about them, that determines whether such events have a negative or positive effect on one's life ,whether they're experienced as opportunity or stress,"

David R. Hawkins, MD, PhD
author, POWER VS. FORCE

Date:

Appointments:

Results/Reports:

Prescriptions:

Things to do:

Thoughts:

Meditation:

I will not accept pain, anger or fear today.

MY CANCER DIARY

"Subtle grades of depression kill more people than all the other diseases of mankind combined, there is no anti-depressant that will cure a depression that's spiritually bases.

David R. Hawkins, MD, PhD
author, POWER VS. FORCE

Date:

Appointments:

Results/Reports:

Prescriptions:

Things to do:

Thoughts:

Meditation:

I will not allow myself to be depressed today.

MY CANCER DIARY

"What stands out about my experience are the relationships I have developed with my caregivers over the years. Let's face it, medicine is medicine, but if there's no relationship I don't think it's quite as effective."

Dorrie Bowden, survivor
Ovarian Cancer
HEALTHLINE MAGAZINE

Date:

Appointments:

Results/Reports:

Prescriptions:

Things to do:

Thoughts:

Meditation:

I am grateful and loving toward my caregivers.

MY CANCER DIARY

"When we have a headache or suffer indigestion, we are quick to look outside for the cause. While the external environment may be harsh and demanding, it can't make us sick. It doesn't determine our attitude. Taking responsibility for who we are is the most healing action we can take."

Karen Casey
author, THE COURSE

Date:

Appointments:

Results/Reports:

Prescriptions:

Things to do:

Thoughts:

Meditation:

I will not accept pain, anger or fear today.

221

MY CANCER DIARY

"Something important occurs when we choose to commit words to paper; our inner voice crystallizes into formed ideas. The alchemical process creates clarity of thought and allows inner wisdom to come through."

Susan Piver
author, THE HARD QUESTIONS FOR AN
AUTHENTIC LIFE

Date:

Appointments:

Results/Reports:

Prescriptions:

Things to do:

Thoughts:

Meditation:

I will write in my journal every day.

MY CANCER DIARY

"The decision to create is the decision to intend. To create healing, you can't have thoughts of illness and anticipate your falling victim to the disease. You can go within and hold an intention that says, "I want to feel good, I intend to feel good. I feel good. I refuse to allow any thoughts of disease or disorder in."

Dr. Wayne W. Dyer
author, THE POWER OF INTENTION

Date:

Appointments:

Results/Reports:

Prescriptions:

Things to do:

Thoughts:

Meditation:

"Eternal Energy, awaken in me conscious will, conscious vitality, conscious health, conscious realization."

Paramahansa Yogananda

MY CANCER DIARY

"When people believe that life is meaningful and that they have a mission to accomplish they are strongly motivated to commit all their inner mind/body resources to help fight illness. That combination sometimes produces medical miracles."

Herbert Benson, MD
Harvard Medical School
co-author, TIMELESS HEALING

Date:

Appointments:

Results/Reports:

Prescriptions:

Things to do:

Thoughts:

Meditation:

"I have now transcended all patterns of illness, I'm free and healthy!

I am now full of radiant health and energy; I am energetic and full of vitality.

I am good to my body, and my body is good to me."

Shakti Gawain, author
CREATIVE VISULIZATION

MY CANCER DIARY

"We've learned that for every effect in our lives, there's a thought pattern that precedes and maintains it. Our consistent thinking patterns create our experiences. Therefore, by changing our thinking patterns, we can change our experiences."

Louise L. Hay,
author, YOU CAN HEAL YOUR
LIFE

Date:

Appointments:

Results/Reports:

Prescriptions:

Things to do:

Thoughts:

Meditation:

With a gentle had I release regret. With acceptance I acknowledge lessons learned. With gratitude I give thanks for the richness of my experience. With a generous heart I share the treasures of my wisdom.

MY CANCER DIARY

"Rather than give relief to the body, give relief to the mind. When the mind is at peace the body is not distressed."

MUMON (1900-1988)

Date:

Appointments:

Results/Reports:

Prescriptions:

Things to do:

Thoughts:

Meditation:

Close your eyes and visualize white healing energy passing through the top of your head down through your body, passing into and through the distressed part of your body. Do not be alarmed if you feel a tingle, just continue and repeat for 5 minutes or more every day.

I feel the warm glow of the healing white energy engulf my bbody.

MY CANCER DIARY

"There is nothing the body suffers which the soul may not profit by."

George Meredith (1828-1909)

Date:

Appointments:

Results/Reports:

Prescriptions:

Things to do:

Thoughts:

Meditation:

Visualize a place where you always felt safe and in a healing space, either from childhood, or even a favorite vacation spot at which you were happy, and at peace. Visit this place in your mind to comfort you when you are feeling badly.

I am safe. I am home.

MY CANCER DIARY

"Miracles do not happen in contradiction to nature, but only in contradiction to that which is known to us of nature."

ST. AGUSTINE (354-430ce)

Date:

Appointments:

Results/Reports:

Prescriptions:

Things to do:

Thoughts:

Meditation:

"Unto this darkness, which beyond light, we pray that we come, and through loss of sight and knowledge may we see and know that which transcends sight and knowledge, by the very fact of not seeing and knowing- for this is the real sight and knowledge"

DIONYSIUS (c.500ce)

MY CANCER DIARY

"Guided imagery was one of the modalities on which, to my great surprise, I had found studies proving beyond a doubt that it could influence recovery rates for patients with cancer."

Candace B. Pert, PhD, behavioral neuroscientist
author,   MOLECULES OF EMOTION

Date:

Appointments:

Results/Reports:

Prescriptions:

Things to do:

Thoughts:

Meditation:

My body is balanced, in perfect harmony with the universe. I give thanks for ever increasing health, beauty, and vitality. I am a radiant expression of God. My mind and my body now manifest divine perfection.

Shakti Gawain
author, Creative Visualization

MY CANCER DIARY

"In my own practice, several cancer patients have recovered completely after being pronounced incurable and given only a few months to live. I didn't think they were miracles; I thought they were proof that the mind can go deep enough to change the very patterns that design the body. It can wipe out mistakes off the blue print and destroy any disease that disturbed the design."

Deepak Chopra, MD
author, QUANTUM HEALING

Date:

Appointments:

Results/Reports:

Prescriptions:

Things to do:

Thoughts:

Meditation:

(Quietly surrender yourself by creating positive thoughts that support your immune system. Love your body and send it loving thoughts that will penetrate you organs and your very cells, making them strong and powerful as they heal. See your body in perfect health every day. Move toward that image.)

I AM HEALTHY. I AM STRONG. I AM WELL!

MY CANCER DIARY

"One of my patients, a 28 year old man, had experienced a complete remission from cancer after receiving a bone marrow transplant, But he hadn't slept for months. He was afraid he would never wake up. Guided imagery gave him a sense of peace that enabled him to release that fear. Soon he was able to get the restorative sleep he needed to stay well."

Mitchell L. Gaynor, MD.
Weil Cornell Medical College
author, HEALING ESSENCE

Date:

Appointments:

Results/Reports:

Prescriptions:

Things to do:

Thoughts:

Meditation:

I am healthy. I am powerful. I am without fear.

MY CANCER DIARY

"Every detail of the belief system that we hold has consequences for better or for worse. It's for this reason that there is no such thing as an incurable or hopeless condition.-somewhere, at some time, somebody has recovered from it."

David R. Hawkins, MD, PhD
author, POWER VS. FORCE

Date:

Appointments:

Results/Reports:

Prescriptions:

Things to do:

Thoughts:

Meditation:

I feel great! I feel wonderful. My body is getting stronger and stronger every day.

MY CANCER DIARY

"Close relationships with friends and family members seem to have significant and highly beneficial effects on the immune system. Studies have linked happiness and positive emotions to longer survival among cancer patients."

Steven Locke, MD
Harvard Medical School
author, THE HEALER WITHIN

Date:

Appointments:

Results/Reports:

Prescriptions:

Things to do:

Thoughts:

Meditation:

When you feel most alone, imagine your good friends gathered around you. They have their healing hands on your shoulder. They are whispering to you that you are very special and very loved. Feel their healing warmth, and their gentle nurturing support,

The healing love of God engulfs me. God is with me and all is well.

MY CANCER DIARY

"One of the things I did to heal myself was to watch very funny movies. That's all we would do was laugh, laugh and laugh. "

Cathy Goodman
Breast Cancer Survivor

Date:

Appointments:

Results/Reports:

Prescriptions:

Things to do:

Thoughts:

Meditation:

Today I remember all the things that made laugh in my life time, and I will laugh and laugh all day.

MY CANCER DIARY

We all come with a built in basic program of healing. It's called "self-healing". You get a wound, it grows back together. You get a bacterial infection; the immune system comes and takes care of those bacteria, and heals it up. The immune system is made to heal itself."

Ben Johnson, MD
author, THE HEALING CODES

Date:

Appointments:

Results/Reports:

Prescriptions:

Things to do:

Thoughts:

Meditation:

I believe in the power of my mind to heal my body. I believe in the power of my spirit to heal my mind. I feel strong. I feel vital. Every day I am getting better and better.

MY CANCER DIARY

"The irony is that our limited perception stops us from seeing these realms which exists right under our three-dimensional noses! Also delighting me, The National Institutes of Health are funding reams of new research on energy therapies-from how Yoga can help insomnia to how Gigong can serve as an adjunct to cancer treatment."

Judith Orloff, MD

author, POSITIVE ENERGY

Date:

Appointments:

Results/Reports:

Prescriptions:

Things to do:

Thoughts:

Meditation:

I know that everything in my life serves a purpose. I will only focus on the things that are positive

And that I need in my life. I will let go of all things I don't need in my life.

MY CANCER DIARY

"As long as the patient is convinced by his symptoms, he is caught up in a reality where "being sick" is the dominant input. The reason why meditation is so important in Ayurveda is because it leads the mind to a "free zone". Until you know that such a place exists, your disease will seem to be taking over completely."

Deepak Chopra, MD,
author, QUANTUM HEALING

Date:

Appointments:

Results/Reports:

Prescriptions:

Things to do:

Thoughts:

Meditation:

Place your hands upon the affected part of your body. Close your eyes and visualize white healing energy passing through head to your arms, to your warm hands. Concentrate the energy and the power of your positive thinking mind down to your warm, sensitive, healing hands.

The healing light of God surrounds me. The healing power of God flows through me.

MY CANCER DIARY

"Consider whence each thing is come, and of what it consists, and into what it changes, and what kind of thing it will be when it has changed, and that it will sustain no harm."

Marcus Aurelius,
Emperor of Rome. AD 121

Date:

Appointments:

Results/Reports:

Prescriptions:

Things to do:

Thoughts:

Meditation:

I now know that awareness is the very first step in healing. I will work toward becoming being more aware each day.

MY CANCER DIARY

"In meditation the mind is held steady and not focused by grim determination, but by its own ability to enter into awareness once we stop distracting it. So how do we try to stop the stream of thinking? The answer is, you don't try. You decide to concentrate on your breathing."

David Fontana, PhD
author, MEDITATION

Date:

Appointments:

Results/Reports:

Prescriptions:

Things to do:

Thoughts:

Meditation:

I will rise above all negative thoughts and physical limitations. I will only focus on my healed strong body and mind.

MY CANCER DIARY

"Time is like a river made up of the events which happen, and a violent stream; for as soon as the thing has been seen, it is carried away, and another comes in its place, and this will be carried away too."

**Marcus Aurelius, Emperor
of Rome (AD 121-180)**

Date:

Appointments:

Results/Reports:

Prescriptions:

Things to do:

Thoughts:

Meditation:

Today I will go with the flow

MY CANCER DIARY

"Many studies and observations through the years have suggested the possible role of emotions in the etiology and course of cancer. There is ample evidence that psychological factors play some role in the genesis and the subsequent course of cancer once it has begun."

John E. Sarno, MD
author, THE MIND BODY PRESCRIPTION

Date:

Appointments:

Results/Reports:

Prescriptions:

Things to do:

Thoughts:

Meditation:

I blame no one for my disease, especially myself. I am one with the power that created me and with the help of this very same power I will transcend all patterns of illness.

MY CANCER DIARY

"At Stanford University, researchers showed Bizzaro comics to people while their brains were monitored by an MRI. They proved that humor stimulates the parts of the brain that use the "feel good chemical dopamine. All the suggestions are that laughter is indeed good for you. So get those convulsions going and chuckle yourself to health."

William Weed
writer, READERS DIGEST

Date:

Appointments:

Results/Reports:

Prescriptions:

Things to do:

Thoughts:

Meditation:

Concentrate on the lives of Bob Hope, Milton Berle, George Burns, and Charlie Chaplin and how long they lived.

I will start seeing the funny side of life and plan to live to a ripe old age.

MY CANCER DIARY

"Happier thoughts lead to essentially happier biochemistry, a happier healthier body. Negative thoughts and stress have been shown to seriously degrade the body and the functioning of the brain, because it's our thoughts and emotions that are continuously reassembling, re-organizing, and re-creating our body."

John Hagelin, PhD
Quantum Physicist

Date:

Appointments:

Results/Reports:

Prescriptions:

Things to do:

Thoughts:

Meditation:

I now release all angry negative feelings. I am willing to feel happy, healthy and strong.

MY CANCER DIARY

"Our doubts and misperceptions, normal in any learning process, trigger the aches and pains we experience. Simply acknowledge this and then allowing our minds to change will in turn, change the way the body feels."

Karen Casey
author, THE COURSE

Date:

Appointments:

Results/Reports:

Prescriptions:

Things to do:

Thoughts:

Meditation:

I now choose to believe in my healing. I have power and authority over my body, my health, my mind and my life.

244

MY CANCER DIARY

"While westerners may consider subtle energy esoteric or New Age, it's been central to many healing traditions for millennia. Therapeutic touch (hands on –healing) has already been shown to accelerate wound healing and the immune system and to relieve pain. At New York's Presbyterian Hospital energy healers have been utilized during open-heart surgery."

Judith Orloff, MD
author, POSITIVE ENERGY

Date:

Appointments:

Results/Reports:

Prescriptions:

Things to do:

Thoughts:

Meditation:

Picture yourself only in perfect health, with a golden healing light around the trouble body area,while touching the area with a warm soothing hand.

"I am a radiant expression of God. My mind and my body now manifest divine perfection"

Shakti Gawain, author
CREATIVE VISUALIZATION

MY CANCER DIARY

"The most important treatment any healer can offer is hope for the health and wellbeing of those who suffer disease or trauma. Lack of faith in the power of Spirit to heal plays a deleterious role in the healing process."

Wayne Dyer, PhD
author, THE POWER OF INTENTION

Date:

Appointments:

Results/Reports:

Prescriptions:

Things to do:

Thoughts:

Meditation:

I trust the power of Spirit and the positive process of life to bring me to my excellent health.

MY CANCER DIARY

"How we react depends upon the world we're reacting to. Who we become, as well as what we see, is determined by perception.-which can be said, simply to create the world."

David R. Hawkins, MD, PhD
author, POWER VS. FORCE

Date:

Appointments:

Results/Reports:

Prescriptions:

Things to do:

Thoughts:

Meditation:

The warm golden divine light within me is healing and creating miracles in my life here and now.

MY CANCER DIARY

"I pulled out a diagram that depicted how there were two chains of nerve bundles located on either side of the spinal cord, each rich with many of the information-carrying peptides. [The Yogi] placed his own chakra (subtle energy center) map over my drawing and together we saw how the two systems overlapped. It was the first time I seriously considered that there might be a connection between my work and the Eastern viewpoint."

Candace Pert, Ph.D. Behavioral Neuroscientist author, MOLECULES OF EMOTION

Date:

Appointments:

Results/Reports:

Prescriptions:

Things to do:

Thoughts:

Meditation:

I am a constant flow of energy living in this body.

MY CANCER DIARY

"The purpose of life is to live it, to taste experience to the utmost, to reach out eagerly and without fear for newer and richer experience."

Eleanor Roosevelt

Date:

Appointments:

Results/Reports:

Prescriptions:

Things to do:

Thoughts:

Meditation:

"My business is not to remake myself, but to make the absolute best of what God made."

Robert Browning

MY CANCER DIARY

"Creativity is present in everyone, all the time-in the way we see, smell, taste, touch and hear the world around us. To be creative is simply to be present in the moment, to feel what is happening around and within us right now. Our creativity is what gives meaning to every moment of our lives"

Susan Piver
author, HARD QUESTIONS FOR
AN AUTHENTIC LIFE

Date:

Appointments:

Results/Reports:

Prescriptions:

Things to do:

Thoughts:

Meditation:

Today I will explore my creativity.

MY CANCER DIARY

"If you look under your depression, you will find anger. Look under your anger, and you will find sadness. And under your sadness is the root of it all, what's really masquerading all the while-fear."

Carolyn Sterns
author, PSYCHIC MASSEUSE

Date:

Appointments:

Results/Reports:

Prescriptions:

Things to do:

Thoughts:

Meditation:

I am afraid of nothing. I release all control to the Great Power of the Universe. I feel at peace with my body and my mine.

MY CANCER DIARY

"Because magic seems so foreign to it, the rational part of our minds is generally quite fearful of the non-rational part....One is lead to believe that magical thinking is an act of healing, and that the most magical minds are therefore the healthiest."

Deepak Chopra, MD
author, UNCONDITIONAL LIFE

Date:

Appointments:

Results/Reports:

Prescriptions:

Things to do:

Thoughts:

Meditation:

I celebrate my body and rejoice in its health. I am strong, and glowing with power.

MY CANCER DIARY

"I rejoice in life for its own sake. Life is not a brief candle to me. It's a sort of splendid torch which I hold up for the moment and make it burn brightly as possible."

George Bernard Shaw

Date:

Appointments:

Results/Reports:

Prescriptions:

Things to do:

Thoughts:

Meditation:

I recognize my magnificent being. Like a glowing torch, I rise high above all my limitations.

MY CANCER DIARY

"That which we persist in doing become easier- not that the nature of the task has changes, but our ability to do has increased."

Ralph Waldo Emerson

Date:

Appointments:

Results/Reports:

Prescriptions:

Things to do:

Thoughts:

Meditation:

I will ask for what I want, again and again and again. I know I will receive what I need most.

MY CANCER DIARY

"We are not human beings having a spiritual experience. We are spiritual beings having a human experience."

Teillard de Chardin, philosopher

Date:

Appointments:

Results/Reports:

Prescriptions:

Things to do:

Thoughts:

Meditation:

My spirit lives in the perfect place at the perfect time. I will always be safe and secure.

MY CANCER DIARY

"All bliss vanishes when the mind takes on suffering; all suffering vanishes when the mind takes on bliss. The reason this must be so is that our inner mirror, unlike one made of glass, actually becomes the image it reflects."

Deepak Chopra, MD
author, UNCONDITIONAL LIFE

Date:

Appointments:

Results/Reports:

Prescriptions:

Things to do:

Thoughts:

Meditation:

I see in my mirror today the image of a strong, healing person. I see the reflection of my healthy face, body and mind.

MY CANCER DIARY

*"To be ready for wholeness, first be fragmented. To be ready for fullness, first be empty.
To be ready for renewal, first be worn out. To be ready for success, first fail."*

**Lao Tzu 6th Century
author, The TAO TE CHING**

Date:

Appointments:

Results/Reports:

Prescriptions:

Things to do:

Thoughts:

Meditation:

I am becoming more and more aware each day. The more aware I become, the more I heal.

I am healing more and more each day.

MY CANCER DIARY

"The greater danger for most of us is not that our aim is too high and we miss it, but that our aim is too low and we reach it."

Michelangelo

Date:

Appointments:

Results/Reports:

Prescriptions:

Things to do:

Thoughts:

Meditation:

I expect perfect health. My expectations of perfect health create my perfect health.

MY CANCER DIARY

"What if you slept? And what if in your sleep you dreamed you went to heaven and there plucked a strange and beautiful flower? And what if when you awoke, you had the flower in your hand?

Samuel Taylor Coleridge (1772-1834)
poet

Date:

Appointments:

Results/Reports:

Prescriptions:

Things to do:

Thoughts:

Meditation:

I choose to dream dreams of health and happiness. It is my divine right to do so.

MY CANCER DIARY

"Today, mind/body interactions are accepted by many in the medical community. Recent studies show that stress-reducing techniques can cause measurable changes in the immune system."

**Medical Consensus Survey of
200 leading cancer experts
PREVENTION MAGAZINE**

Date:

Appointments:

Results/Reports:

Prescriptions:

Things to do:

Thoughts:

Meditation:

**I expect my life to be stress free, and filled with the joy of living.
I am grateful for all the loving things that are given to me.**

MY CANCER DIARY

"Every detail of the belief system that we hold has consequences for better or for worst. It's for this reason that there's no such thing as an incurable disease or hopeless condition-somewhere, at some time, somebody has recovered from it through the process describe."

David R. Hawkins, MD, PhD
author, POWER VS. FORCE

Date:

Appointments:

Results/Reports:

Prescriptions:

Things to do:

Thoughts:

Meditation:

 I believe in my power to heal myself,

MY CANCER DIARY

"All the evidence suggests that for the most people chronic pain is a stress related disorder, just like ulcers. "

Dr. John Loeser, pain expert
University of Washington

Date:

Appointments:

Results/Reports:

Prescriptions:

Things to do:

Thoughts:

Meditation:

Today I will think of all the people I love, and that love me.

MY CANCER DIARY

"Maybe it's not really pain but a metaphor for anxiety and depression or spiritual suffering. We use pain for physical distress, and sometimes people don't make a distinction very well"

Elisabeth Rosenthal,
writer "Chronic Pain", NEW YORK TIMES

Date:

Appointments:

Results/Reports:

Prescriptions:

Things to do:

Thoughts:

Meditation:

I always think positive. I expect good experiences. I deserve good experiences. Life brings me good experiences.

MY CANCER DIARY

"A disease process is evidence that something is amiss in the working of the mind, and that's where the power to effect change resides."

David R. Hawkins, MD, PhD
author, POWER VS. FORCE

Date:

Appointments:

Results/Reports:

Prescriptions:

Things to do:

Thoughts:

Meditation:

I will only accept positive thoughts today.

MY CANCER DIARY

"The reason many psychological factors have been related to cancer is that they all induce internal rage. Work must be done on the source of the rage, not the rage itself."

John E. Sarno, MD
author, The Mindbody Prescription

Date:

Appointments:

Results/Reports:

Prescriptions:

Things to do:

Thoughts:

Meditation:

The past has no power over me. I know the past is over and today I only live in the present.

MY CANCER DIARY

"Round up all the people who are making you miserable and bring them to me. I will treat them as a counselor, and you will get better."

Wayne Dyer, PhD
author, THE POWER OF INTENTION

Date:

Appointments:

Results/Reports:

Prescriptions:

Things to do:

Thoughts:

Meditation:

I am independent, and not at the mercy of other peoples poor behavior. The road to love is forgiveness. I will forgive and travel on.

MY CANCER DIARY

"The body is a reflection of the spirit in its physical expression, and its problems are the dramatization of the struggles of the spirit that gives life. A belief that we ascribe "out there" has its effect; in here."

David R. Hawkins, MD, PhD
author, POWER VS. FORCE

Date:

Appointments:

Results/Reports:

Prescriptions:

Things to do:

Thoughts:

Meditation:

I will fix "out there" by working "in here."

MY CANCER DIARY

"Most people don't recognize that the mind constantly chatters. And yet that chatter winds up being the force that that drives us much of the day, in terms of what we do, what we react to and what we feel. Meditation is a way of looking deeply into the chatter of the mind and body, and becoming more aware of patterns."

Jon Karat-Zinn, PhD
author, FULL CATASTROPHE LIVING

Date:

Appointments:

Results/Reports:

Prescriptions:

Things to do:

Thoughts:

Meditation:

I believe in perfect health. I believe in a healthy body. I believe in a healthy mind.

MY CANCER DIARY

"Cancer made me appreciate all that I have so much more. It taught me to enjoy every moment and to never, ever give up"

Ned Burns, survivor
Non-Hodgkin's lymphoma
HEALTHLINE MAGAZINE

Date:

Appointments:

Results/Reports:

Prescriptions:

Things to do:

Thoughts:

Meditation:

I will rise above my doubt and enjoy every minute of day.

MY CANCER DIARY

"At first I was scared and I didn't know how I was going to make it. I didn't think I was that strong. Then it struck me, even if only one per cent of people like me live, why couldn't I be in that one per cent?"

Eva Dupuy, survivor
Lung Cancer
HEALTHLINE MAGAZINE

Date:

Appointments:

Results/Reports:

Prescriptions:

Things to do:

Thoughts:

Meditation:

I am fearless. I am indestructible. I am a survivor.

MY CANCER DIARY

"My cancer taught me several important lessons. For one it taught me patience, because even though I decided I would be okay, I still had to go through all my treatments. It also taught me how to accept help from others. I had always been the person that helped everyone else; now it was their turn to be strong for me, and I think that helped all of us through the experience."

Valerie Lee, survivor
Breast Cancer
HEALTHLINE MAGAZINE

Date:

Appointments:

Results/Reports:

Prescriptions:

Things to do:

Thoughts:

Meditation:

I am patient, and I will endure all it takes on my way to full recovering.

MY CANCER DIARY

"I get up every morning and thank the person above that I am still alive. And I tell anyone, don't give up hope. It is truly remarkable, even with cancer; I've not missed a step in living my life."

Robert Hong, survivor
Stage 4 Colon Cancer
HEALTHLINE MAGAZINE

Date:

Appointments:

Results/Reports:

Prescriptions:

Things to do:

Thoughts:

Meditation:

Thank you for my life .Thank you for all my blessings. Thank you for this wonderful day.

MY CANCER DIARY

"It's possible that if you live with fear, which many people do, day after day, month after month, the mechanisms that pump these natural killer cells [cancer fighting cells] into our bloodstream or increase their activity they get depleted over time. "

Margaret Kemmeny, PhD
Psychologist, University of Los Angeles

Date:

Appointments:

Results/Reports:

Prescriptions:

Things to do:

Thoughts:

Meditation:

I am fearless. I am powerful. I am a survivor.

MY CANCER DIARY

"Emotional fluctuations and emotional status directly influence the probability that the organism will get sick or be well."

**Candace Pert, PhD, behavioral neuroscientist
author, MOLECULES OF EMOTION**

Date:

Appointments:

Results/Reports:

Prescriptions:

Things to do:

Thoughts:

Meditation:

I am in full control of my mind, my emotions and my body.

MY CANCER DIARY

"If one person is saved one major operation by learning how to self-regulate using mind/body techniques, we've paid for most of the other patients in the clinic for the entire year."

Jon Kabat-Zinn, PhD
author, FULL CATASROPHE LIVING

Date:

Appointments:

Results/Reports:

Prescriptions:

Things to do:

Thoughts:

Meditation:

I control my life, my mind my health.

MY CANCER DIARY

"There is no question that your body and your mind tied together can help fight infection. Part of it is caused by lack of self-care, and I think part of it is a kind of turn off of the immune system."

Ron Anderson, MD
author, MEDICAL APERRTHEID

Date:

Appointments:

Results/Reports:

Prescriptions:

Things to do:

Thoughts:

Meditation:

What I believe I can achieve. What I conceive, I will receive.

MY CANCER DIARY

"When you find positive meaning in every aspect of your life and start to realize that there is a greater force operating, you begin to develop the spirituality essential for true health."

Elliot Dacher, M. D.
author, WHOLE HEALING

Date:

Appointments:

Results/Reports:

Prescriptions:

Things to do:

Thoughts:

Meditation:

I recognize, respect and am in cooperation with a greater force without and within.

MY CANCER DIARY

"There is a growing body of evidence, much of it European that suggests that emotional history is extremely important in things like the incidence of cancer."

Candace Pert, PhD, behavioral neuroscientist
author, MOLECULES OF EMOTION

Date:

Appointments:

Results/Reports:

Prescriptions:

Things to do:

Thoughts:

Meditation:

Today I will heal myself by letting go of all past grudges and forgiving others.

MY CANCER DIARY

"No condition is anything more than a teaching tool. Whenever we learn something new, it changes ever so slightly how we view everything in our lives"

Karen Casey
author, THE COURSE

Date:

Appointments:

Results/Reports:

Prescriptions:

Things to do:

Thoughts:

Meditation:

My mind and my body are a peace today. I choose to feel great and be well today.

MY CANCER DIARY

"It's possible that during certain psychological states like severe unhappiness, you have changes in the brain which result in changes in hormone levels. Those hormones, circulating throughout the bloodstream over the course of the day, then have impact on our immune system."

Margaret Kemeny, PhD
Psychiatry Dept., UCLA

Date:

Appointments:

Results/Reports:

Prescriptions:

Things to do:

Thoughts:

Meditation:

Today I will look inside myself for true happiness.

MY CANCER DIARY

"They realized that the air in the mine would only last a limited amount of hours. As it turned out only one man had a watch, and he began to announce the time while the other men anxiously awaited rescue. To sustain hope in the others he did not announce the right time. He called out one hour when in fact two hours had passed. Six days later a rescue team found the trapped miners all alive with one exception-the man with the watch."

Deepak Chopra, MD
author, UNCONDITIONAL LIFE

Date:

Appointments:

Results/Reports:

Prescriptions:

Things to do:

Thoughts:

Meditation:

I am patient. I am not time bound. I believe.

MY CANCER DIARY

"We are raised to think of miracles as unique, rare occurrences that few people deserve. Our familiarity with miracles is limited; particularly if we define them as dramatic healings…What do we need to make a miracle? Willingness. A change of mind will result in a miracle every time…"

Karen Casey
author, THE COURSE

Date:

Appointments:

Results/Reports:

Prescriptions:

Things to do:

Thoughts:

Meditation:

What I see outside, I produced inside.

MY CANCER DIARY

"Explore everything around you, penetrate to the further limits of human knowledge, and always you will come up with something inexplicable in the end. It is called life."

Albert Schweitzer

Date:

Appointments:

Results/Reports:

Prescriptions:

Things to do:

Thoughts:

Meditation:

I will take this time to learn, to explore and to grow.

MY CANCER DIARY

"An illness is a localized form of unease (as the term disease implies), and it is not surprising that, for many people, a much broader unease underlies it,"

Deepak Chopra, MD
author, UNCONDITIONAL LIFE

Date:

Appointments:

Results/Reports:

Prescriptions:

Things to do:

Thoughts:

Meditation:

I will find peace and comfort today.

MY CANCER DIARY

"We have all heard a story of someone being cured of cancer. Wouldn't that be a miracle in the body? Some might argue yes, however, many would say a change in the body has to be precipitated by a change in the mind."

Karen Casey
author, THE COURSE

Date:

Appointments:

Results/Reports:

Prescriptions:

Things to do:

Thoughts:

Meditation:

I will monitor my minds work today. What I think is all powerful.

MY CANCER DIARY

"When we say we feel a certain way, our mood is always produced by one brain chemical or another- There is no state of mind without a biochemical foundation."

Deepak Chopra, MD
author, UNCONDITIONAL LIFE

Date:

Appointments:

Results/Reports:

Prescriptions:

Things to do:

Thoughts:

Meditation:

I control my thoughts. I control my brain chemicals. I control my feelings.

MY CANCER DIARY

"The same stream of life that runs through my veins night and day runs through the world and dances in rhythmic measures. It is the same life that shoots in joy through the dust of the earth in numberless blades of grass and breaks into tumultuous waves of leaves and flowers."

Tagore, poet

Date:

Appointments:

Results/Reports:

Prescriptions:

Things to do:

Thoughts:

Meditation:

I am one with the universe. The universe always provides.

MY CANCER DIARY

"And now here is my secret. A very simple secret; it is only with the heart that one can see rightly; what is essential is invisible to the eye."

Antoine de Saint-Exupery

Date:

Appointments:

Results/Reports:

Prescriptions:

Things to do:

Thoughts:

Meditation:

I only see with my heart.

MY CANCER DIARY

"If I had my life to live over, I would start barefoot earlier in the spring and stay that way later in the fall. I would go to more dances. I would ride more merry-go-rounds. I would pick more daisies."

Nadine Stair, age 85

Date:

Appointments:

Results/Reports:

Prescriptions:

Things to do:

Thoughts:

Meditation:

I will live my life to the fullest. Today I will dance barefoot like nobody is watching.

MY CANCER DIARY

"If you bite into a lemon, the juice instantly makes your mouth water as salivary glands under your tongue start secreting two digestive enzymes, but what happens if you merely visualize a lemon, or think the word lemon three times to yourself? Again the mouth waters and the same salivary enzymes are produced eve thought there is nothing to digest. The message sent to the brain is more important than the presence of actual food. Words and images function just as well as the "real" molecules to trigger the ongoing process of life.

Deepak Chopra, MD
author, AGELESS BODY, TIMELESS MIND

Date:

Appointments:

Results/Reports:

Prescriptions:

Things to do:

Thoughts:

Meditation:

I will take control of my body by taking control of my words and images.

MY CANCER DIARY

"When we have a headache or suffer indigestion, we are quick to look outside for the cause. While the external environment may be harsh and demanding, it can't make us sick. It doesn't determine our attitude. Taking responsibility for who we are is the most healing action we can take."

Karen Casey
author, THE COURSE

Date:

Appointments:

Results/Reports:

Prescriptions:

Things to do:

Thoughts:

Meditation:

I will not accept pain, anger or fear today.

MY CANCER DIARY

"Treating an illness as a physical process only doesn't correct the origin of the dysfunction, and covers it up instead of curing it. It's possible for a lifelong affliction to heal rapidly with the mere shift of attitude; but though this shift may seem to occur in a split second, it may in actuality take years of inner preparation."

David R. Hawkins, MD, PhD
author, POWER VS. FORCE

Date:

Appointments:

Results/Reports:

Prescriptions:

Things to do:

Thoughts:

Meditation:

I always have a positive attitude about life.

MY CANCER DIARY

"Belief creates biology."

Norman Cousins, cancer survivor
author, ANATOMY OF AN ILLNESS

Date:

Appointments:

Results/Reports:

Prescriptions:

Things to do:

Thoughts:

Meditation:

I believe I can heal. I believe I am healing. I believe I am healed.

MY CANCER DIARY

"Watching a humorous video (in this case a comedian) reduced levels of adrenaline and cortisol in the blood stream. These and other substances that suppress immunity are produced by the body in great quantities during times of stress."

Loma Linda University Study

Date:

Appointments:

Results/Reports:

Prescriptions:

Things to do:

Thoughts:

Meditation:

I will not stress today.

MY CANCER DIARY

"Elderly people received training in progressive muscle relaxation. The subjects had significantly more natural killer cells, a type of immunity that protects against viral illness and cancer, in their blood streams after training than they did before. However, it is cautioned that patients who wish to use these techniques should not abandon their conventional treatments."

Ohio University Study

Date:

Appointments:

Results/Reports:

Prescriptions:

Things to do:

Thoughts:

Meditation:

Today I will work on relaxing my body.

MY CANCER DIARY

"We all suffer fears, painful memories and disappointments. We forget who we truly are as we struggle to meet unrealistic expectations, and condemn those around us who fail to meet our expectations of them. We push these feeling aside, but they take their toll."

Mitchell L. Gaynor, MD, cancer specialist
author, HEALING ESSENCE

Date:

Appointments:

Results/Reports:

Prescriptions:

Things to do:

Thoughts:

Meditation:

I will let go of all past negative feelings and regrets.

MY CANCER DIARY

"Medical researchers now recognize that it is impossible to separate your mind's health from your body's health. What you believe, think, or feel will affect your body in the short and the long term, and a growing number of experts suspect that you use your mind not only to ward off illnesses, but also to help heal yourself when you get sick."

Elliot Dacher, MD
author, WHOLE HEALING

Date:

Appointments:

Results/Reports:

Prescriptions:

Things to do:

Thoughts:

Meditation:

When I control my mind, I control my body.

MY CANCER DIARY

"Symptoms of illnesses may be more than signs of a physical problem. Often they are a signal that something is out of sync in your life, that some aspect of your approach to life needs changing."

Elliot Dasher, MD
author; WHOLE HEALING

Date:

Appointments:

Results/Reports:

Prescriptions:

Things to do:

Thoughts:

Meditation:

Today I will listen to my body. I will work to understand what it is trying to tell me.

MY CANCER DIARY

"Finding meaning in one's life, studies show, is an essential part of good health. While it is easy to discover meaning in the positive aspects of life, it is difficult to find meaning and purpose in life's difficulties. Rather than feeling powerless or angry, ask, Is there something I can learn from this"?

Elliot Dacher, MD
author, WHOLE HEALING

Date:

Appointments:

Results/Reports:

Prescriptions:

Things to do:

Thoughts:

Meditation:

I will search for meaning in all aspects of my life.

MY CANCER DIARY

"Just as your body needs sleep for renewal and optimum health, your mind needs periods of quiet and solitude. A quiet mind reveals important things about life, changes you may need to make for a healthier, richer lifestyle. A period of solitude "recharges the brain and the body."

**Elliot Dacher, MD
author, WHOLE HEALING**

Date:

Appointments:

Results/Reports:

Prescriptions:

Things to do:

Thoughts:

Meditation:

Today I will learn to be still.

MY CANCER DIARY

"When you learn to listen to and trust the messages your body sends, you will be taking an important step toward achieving optimal health."

Elliot Dacher, MD
author, WHOLE HEALING

Date:

Appointments:

Results/Reports:

Prescriptions:

Things to do:

Thoughts:

Meditation:

I will not accept pain, anger or fear today.

MY CANCER DIARY

"People who dislike what they do often get sick as a result of inevitable psychological stress. I have seen many cancer patients suddenly quit their jobs and start doing what they always wanted to do. Many of these individuals lived longer, healthier lives."

Bernie Siegel, MD
author, HOW TO LIVE BETWEEN OFFICE VISITS

Date:

Appointments:

Results/Reports:

Prescriptions:

Things to do:

Thoughts:

Meditation:

I will do what I love, and love what I do for the rest of my life.

MY CANCER DIARY

"You have an absolute right to ask for help whenever you need it. This goes for practical dad-to-day items like food and transportation, as well as for emotional support when you're feeling sad or lonely."

Bernie Siegel, MD
author, HOW TO LIVE BETWEEN OFFICE VISITS

Date:

Appointments:

Results/Reports:

Prescriptions:

Things to do:

Thoughts:

Meditation:

I will ask for help whenever I need it.

MY CANCER DIARY

"Gratitude unlocks the fullness of life. It turns what we have into enough, and more. It turns denial into acceptance, chaos into order, and confusion into clarity. It can turn a meal into a feast, a house into a home, a stranger into a friend. Gratitude makes sense of our past, brings peace for today and creates a vision for tomorrow."

Melody Beattie
author, THE LANGUAGE OF LETTING GO

Date:

Appointments:

Results/Reports:

Prescriptions:

Things to do:

Thoughts:

Meditation:

Thank you for all my blessings, and thank you for this day.

MY CANCER DIARY

"I like living. I have sometimes been wildly, despairingly, acutely miserable, racked with sorrow, but through it all I still know quite certainly that just to be alive is a grand thing."

Agatha Christie

Date:

Appointments:

Results/Reports:

Prescriptions:

Things to do:

Thoughts:

Meditation:

I will not accept pain, anger or fear today.

MY CANCER DIARY

"When we have a headache or suffer indigestion, we are quick to look outside for the cause. While the external environment may be harsh and demanding, it can't make us sick. It doesn't determine our attitude. Taking responsibility for who we are is the most healing action we can take."

Karen Casey
author, THE COURSE

Date:

Appointments:

Results/Reports:

Prescriptions:

Things to do:

Thoughts:

Meditation:

My life is getting better and better each day.

MY CANCER DIARY

"I can't believe that the inscrutable universe turns on an axis of suffering: surely the strange beauty of the world must somewhere rest on pure joy."

Louis Bogan

Date:

Appointments:

Results/Reports:

Prescriptions:

Things to do:

Thoughts:

Meditation:

Today I will find my joy.

MY CANCER DIARY

"Bless a thing and it will bless you. Curse it and it will curse you...If you bless a situation, it has no power to hurt you, and if it is troublesome for a time, it will gradually fade out, if you sincerely bless it."

Emmet Fox

Date:

Appointments:

Results/Reports:

Prescriptions:

Things to do:

Thoughts:

Meditation:

I bless my life and my circumstances each day.

MY CANCER DIARY

"Grace strikes us when we are in great pain and restlessness...Sometimes at that moment a wave of light breaks into our darkness, and it is as though a voice were saying: You are accepted.

Paul Johannes Tillich

Date:

Appointments:

Results/Reports:

Prescriptions:

Things to do:

Thoughts:

Meditation:

Today I will wait for the healing forces of the universe to do their work with patience and grace.

MY CANCER DIARY

"Learn to get in touch with the silence within yourself and know that everything in this life has a purpose."

Elisabeth Kubler-Ross, psychiatrist

Date:

Appointments:

Results/Reports:

Prescriptions:

Things to do:

Thoughts:

Meditation:

I will allow myself quiet moments each day to restore my sense of purpose.

MY CANCER DIARY

"You must have a room or a certain hour of the day or so, where you do not know what was in the morning paper...a place where you can simply experience and bring forth what you are and what you might be...At first you may find nothing's happening...But if you have a sacred place and use it, take advantage of it, something will happen."

Joseph Campbell
author, THE POWER OF MYTH

Date:

Appointments:

Results/Reports:

Prescriptions:

Things to do:

Thoughts:

Meditation:

I am in my sacred place waiting patiently.

311

MY CANCER DIARY

"Meditation is simply about being yourself ,and knowing about who that is. It is about coming to realize that you are on a path whether you like it or not, namely the path of life."

**Jon Kabat-Zinn
author, FULL CATASTROPHE LIVING**

Date:

Appointments:

Results/Reports:

Prescriptions:

Things to do:

Thoughts:

Meditation:

I will take time each day to know myself.

MY CANCER DIARY

"Inside myself is a place where I live all alone and that's where you renew your springs that never dry up."

Pearl S. Buck
author, THE GOOD EARTH

Date:

Appointments:

Results/Reports:

Prescriptions:

Things to do:

Thoughts:

Meditation:

I am not alone; I am in my special place.

MY CANCER DIARY

"The body is a sacred garment. It's you first and your last garment; it is what you enter life in and what you depart life with, and it should be treated with honor."

Martha Graham, dancer

Date:

Appointments:

Results/Reports:

Prescriptions:

Things to do:

Thoughts:

Meditation:

Today I will exercise as best I can and treat my body with respect and honor.

MY CANCER DIARY

"The body must be nourished, physically, emotional and spiritually. We're spiritually starved in this culture- not underfed but undernourished."

Carol Hornig, nutritionist

Date:

Appointments:

Results/Reports:

Prescriptions:

Things to do:

Thoughts:

Meditation:

Today I will nourish my mind, my spirit and my body.

MY CANCER DIARY

"Today a new sun rises for me; everything lives, everything is animated, everything seems to speak to me of my passion, everything invites me to cherish it."

Anne De Lenclos, survivor
Breast Cancer
HEALTHLINE MAGAZINE

Date:

Appointments:

Results/Reports:

Prescriptions:

Things to do:

Thoughts:

Meditation:

Today I will cherish everything I see and hear and touch.

MY CANCER DIARY

"All you need is deep within you waiting to unfold and reveal itself. All you have to do is be still and take time to seek for what is within, and you will surely find it."

Eileen Caddy
author, OPENING DOORS WITHIN

Date:

Appointments:

Results/Reports:

Prescriptions:

Things to do:

Thoughts:

Meditation:

Today I will search my soul and find what I need.

MY CANCER DIARY

"Difficult times have helped me to understand better than before how infinitely rich and beautiful life is in every way and that so many things that one goes worrying about are of no importance."

Isak Dinesen
author, OUT OF AFRICA

Date:

Appointments:

Results/Reports:

Prescriptions:

Things to do:

Thoughts:

Meditation:

Today is beautiful, and I am part of this day.

MY CANCER DIARY

"Stories are medicine...They have such power; they do not require that we do, be, act anything-we need only listen. The remedies for repair and reclamation of any psychic drive are contained in stories."

Clarrissa Pinkola Estes, poet

Date:

Appointments:

Results/Reports:

Prescriptions:

Things to do:

Thoughts:

Meditation:

Today I will listen to others and I will learn.

MY CANCER DIARY

"The inner experience of meditation can be had without any kind of forced discipline. The outer trappings-how one sits, breathes, dresses, and so forth- are really irrelevant."

Deepak Chopra, MD
author, UNCONDITIONAL LIFE

Date:

Appointments:

Results/Reports:

Prescriptions:

Things to do:

Thoughts:

Meditation:

I will sit quietly and do nothing, not even think.

MY CANCER DIARY

"You gain strength, courage and confidence by every experience in which you really stop to look fear in the face...You must do the thing you cannot do."

Eleanor Roosevelt

Date:

Appointments:

Results/Reports:

Prescriptions:

Things to do:

Thoughts:

Meditation:

"Eternal Energy, awaken in me conscious will, conscious vitality, conscious health, conscious realization."

Paramahansa Yogananda

MY CANCER DIARY

"No matter what you are going through or how difficult it may seem, you can remain standing on the inside. It may take courage. It will definitely take determination, but you can do it if you decide to do so. You must act on your will, not just your emotions."

Joel Osteen, pastor
author, YOUR BEST LIFE NOW

Date:

Appointments:

Results/Reports:

Prescriptions:

Things to do:

Thoughts:

Meditation:

I will always be standing strong on the inside.

MY CANCER DIARY

"Let me remember that each life must follow its own course, and that what happens to other people has absolutely nothing to do with what happens to me."

Marjorie Holmes
author, TWO FROM GALILEE

Date:

Appointments:

Results/Reports:

Prescriptions:

Things to do:

Thoughts:

Meditation:

"I have now transcended all patterns of illness, I'm free and healthy!

Shakti Gawain, author
CREATIVE VISULIZATION

MY CANCER DIARY

"God answers sharp and sudden on some prayers, and thrusts the thing we have prayed for in our face, a gauntlet with a gift in it. "

Elizabeth Barrett Browning

Date:

Appointments:

Results/Reports:

Prescriptions:

Things to do:

Thoughts:

Meditation:

I am thankful for the gift of each day.

MY CANCER DIARY

"There are only two ways to live your life. One is as though nothing is a miracle. The other is as though everything is a miracle."

Albert Einstein

Date:

Appointments:

Results/Reports:

Prescriptions:

Things to do:

Thoughts:

Meditation:

My days are filled with miracles.

MY CANCER DIARY

"We all have angels guiding us…They look after us. They heal us, touch us, and comfort us with invisible warm hands…What will bring their help? Asking. Giving thanks."

Sophy Burnham
author, THE ECSTATIC JOURNEY

Date:

Appointments:

Results/Reports:

Prescriptions:

Things to do:

Thoughts:

Meditation:

I am asking for healing. I am thankful for my life.

MY CANCER DIARY

"Illness is the doctor we pay most heed; to kindness, to knowledge, we make promises only; pain we obey."

Marcel Proust

Date:

Appointments:

Results/Reports:

Prescriptions:

Things to do:

Thoughts:

Meditation:

As I send out positive thoughts, the universe will respond in kind.

MY CANCER DIARY

"Live in each season as it passes; breathe air, drink the drink, taste the fruit, and resign yourself to the influence of each day. Let them be your only diet drink and botanical medicines."

Henry David Thoreau

Date:

Appointments:

Results/Reports:

Prescriptions:

Things to do:

Thoughts:

Meditation:

What a beautiful day. The sun rises and I know I am part of that sun.

MY CANCER DIARY

"We can have anything we want if we want it desperately enough. You must want it with an exuberance that erupts through your skin and joins the energy that created the world."

Sheila Graham

Date:

Appointments:

Results/Reports:

Prescriptions:

Things to do:

Thoughts:

Meditation:

I see my body in perfect health every day. I move toward that image.

MY CANCER DIARY

"In every pain let this thought be present, that there is no dishonor in it, nor does it make the governing intelligence worse, for it does not damage the intelligence....When then thou art discontented about any of these things say to thyself, thou art yielding to the pain."

Marcus Aurelius, Emperor of Rome, AD 161

Date:

Appointments:

Results/Reports:

Prescriptions:

Things to do:

Thoughts:

Meditation:

I am willing to pursue knowledge. I heal through what I learn.

MY CANCER DIARY

"We say the body isn't real and then proceed to affect it by the mind. How can this be? What we mean when we say the body isn't real is that it reflects what the mind projects. It doesn't exist independently."

Karen Casey
author THE COURSE

Date:

Appointments:

Results/Reports:

Prescriptions:

Things to do:

Thoughts:

Meditation:

I feel great! I feel wonderful. My body is getting stronger and stronger every day.

MY CANCER DIARY

"We must guard against putting ourselves down when we manifest illness of any kind. While it's true that right-mindedness can prevent sickness, we're merely students, not avatars, and we're still learning about our minds power as we travel this path."

Karen Casey
author THE COURSE

Date:

Appointments:

Results/Reports:

Prescriptions:

Things to do:

Thoughts:

Meditation:

I truly believed in my heart that I am already healed.

MY CANCER DIARY

"When ignorant people hear about it they laugh out loud! By this very laughter we know its authenticity."

Lao Tzu
TAO TE CHING

Date:

Appointments:

Results/Reports:

Prescriptions:

Things to do:

Thoughts:

Meditation:

I believe in the power of my mind to heal my body. I believe in the power of my spirit to heal my mind. I feel strong. I feel vital. Every day I am getting better and better.

MY CANCER DIARY

"Let me remember that each life must follow its own coursed, and that what happens to others people has absolutely nothing to do with what happens to me."

Majorie Holmes
author, TWO FROM GALILEE

Date:

Appointments:

Results/Reports:

Prescriptions:

Things to do:

Thoughts:

Meditation:

I know that everything in my life serves a purpose for me, and I will not compare myself to others.

MY CANCER DIARY

"There are only hints and guesses, hints followed by guesses, and the rest is prayer, observance, thoughts and action."

T.S. Eliot

Date:

Appointments:

Results/Reports:

Prescriptions:

Things to do:

Thoughts:

Meditation:

I will only think positive. I will only act positive.

MY CANCER DIARY

"First we have to believe, and then we believe."

G. C. Lichtenberg, scientist

Date:

Appointments:

Results/Reports:

Prescriptions:

Things to do:

Thoughts:

Meditation:

I now know that belief is a step in healing. I believe I am healed.

MY CANCER DIARY

"Gratitude makes sense of our past, brings peace for today, and creates a vision for tomorrow"

Melody Beatie
author, THE LANGUAGE OF LETTING GO

Date:

Appointments:

Results/Reports:

Prescriptions:

Things to do:

Thoughts:

Meditation:

I am grateful for today's blessings and tomorrow's healing.

MY CANCER DIARY

"We must be willing to get rid of the life we've planned, so as to have the life that is waiting for us."

Joseph Campbell
author, THE POWER OF MYTH

Date:

Appointments:

Results/Reports:

Prescriptions:

Things to do:

Thoughts:

Meditation:

I am open and ready for the new life that awaits me.

MY CANCER DIARY

"The mind is like a pond. On the surface you see all the disturbances, yet the surface is only a fraction of the pond, it is in the depth below the surface, where there is stillness that you come to know the true essence of the pond, as well as your own mind."

Wayne Dyer, PhD
author, WISDOM OF THE AGES

Date:

Appointments:

Results/Reports:

Prescriptions:

Things to do:

Thoughts:

Meditation:

Today I will explore the silence.

MY CANCER DIARY

"Man is disturbed not by things that happen, but by his opinion of the things that happen."

Epictetus, philosopher (55-135)

Date:

Appointments:

Results/Reports:

Prescriptions:

Things to do:

Thoughts:

Meditation:

Nothing disturbs me. Things are as they should be.

MY CANCER DIARY

"A life time is not what's between the moments of birth and death. A life time is one moment between my two little breaths; the present, the here, the now. That's all the life I get, I live each moment full. In kindness, in peace, without regret,"

Chade-Meng Tan, motivational speaker

Date:

Appointments:

Results/Reports:

Prescriptions:

Things to do:

Thoughts:

Meditation:

I now choose to live every moment in the now.

MY CANCER DIARY

"When I begin to sit with dawn in solitude, I begin to live. It makes me treasure every single moment of life."

Gloria Vanderbilt, designer

Date:

Appointments:

Results/Reports:

Prescriptions:

Things to do:

Thoughts:

Meditation:

Today is a good day to be alive.

MY CANCER DIARY

"When your thoughts have been running in a certain pattern for a long period of time, it's as though you have been digging a deep riverbed, and the water can flow only in one direction. With every pessimistic thought, you dig that river a little bit deeper... Fortunately, it's possible to dig a new river, one going in a positive direction. The way to do it is one thought at a time"

Joel Osteen, pastor
author, YOUR BEST LIFE NOW

Date:

Appointments:

Results/Reports:

Prescriptions:

Things to do:

Thoughts:

Meditation:

Today I will reverse all negative thoughts into positive affirmations.

MY CANCER DIARY

"Happy the man, and happy he alone, he who can call today his own: He who, secure within, can say: tomorrow do thy worst, for I have lived today."

John Dryden, poet

Date:

Appointments:

Results/Reports:

Prescriptions:

Things to do:

Thoughts:

Meditation:

Today is mine.

MY CANCER DIARY

"Satisfaction lies in the effort, not the attainment. Full effort is full victory."

Mahatma Ghandi   (1869-1948)

Date:

Appointments:

Results/Reports:

Prescriptions:

Things to do:

Thoughts:

Meditation:

Today I will make the effort. I will succeed. Today I will heal.

MY CANCER DIARY

"The real voyage of discovery consists not in seeking new landscapes, but in having new eye."

Marcel Proust

Date:

Appointments:

Results/Reports:

Prescriptions:

Things to do:

Thoughts:

Meditation:

I see my healing.

MY CANCER DIARY

"My business is not to remake myself, but to make the absolute best of what God made."

Robert Browning

Date:

Appointments:

Results/Reports:

Prescriptions:

Things to do:

Thoughts:

Meditation:

I am more courageous every day.

MY CANCER DIARY

"The earth seems to rest in silent meditation; and the waters and the sky and the heavens seem all to be in meditation. On earth, those that achieve greatness, they do so through concentration."

THE UPANISHADS

Date:

Appointments:

Results/Reports:

Prescriptions:

Things to do:

Thoughts:

Meditation:

My mind is quiet. My mind is focused.

MY CANCER DIARY

"Find a place inside where there is joy, and the joy will burn out the pain."

Joseph Campbell
author, THE POWER OF MYTH

Date:

Appointments:

Results/Reports:

Prescriptions:

Things to do:

Thoughts:

Meditation:

I remind myself that I have joy within.

MY CANCER DIARY

"There is a hidden strength within me to overcome all obstacles and temptations. I will bring forth that indomitable power and energy."

Paramahanda Yogananda

Date:

Appointments:

Results/Reports:

Prescriptions:

Things to do:

Thoughts:

Meditation:

My energy and power live within. I will bring it forth.

MY CANCER DIARY

"Open the windows of calmness and you will find a sudden burst of joy within your very self. The joyous rays of the soul may be perceived if you interiorize your attention."

Paramahanda Yogananda

Date:

Appointments:

Results/Reports:

Prescriptions:

Things to do:

Thoughts:

Meditation:

Today I will look within to see the reflection of my joy.

MY CANCER DIARY

"Calm in quietude is not real calm. When you can be calm in the midst of activity, this is the true state of nature. Happiness in comfort is not real happiness. When you are happy in the midst of hardship, then you see the true potential of the mind."

Huanchu Daoren

Date:

Appointments:

Results/Reports:

Prescriptions:

Things to do:

Thoughts:

Meditation:

I am becoming more calm each day. The more calm I become, the more happy I become.

The more happy I become, the more healthy I become.

MY CANCER DIARY

"We are not our feelings. We are not our moods. We are not even our thoughts. The very fact that we can think about these things separates us from them. Self-awareness enables us to stand apart and examine even the way we 'see' ourselves."

Stephen R. Covey

author, 7 HABITS OF HIGHLY EFFECTIVE PEOPLE

Date:

Appointments:

Results/Reports:

Prescriptions:

Things to do:

Thoughts:

Meditation:

I choose perfect health as my natural state of being.

MY CANCER DIARY

"What you say in the midst of your difficulties will have a great impact on how long you have to stay in those situations."

Joel Osteen, pastor
author, YOUR BEST LIFE NOW

Date:

Appointments:

Results/Reports:

Prescriptions:

Things to do:

Thoughts:

Meditation:

I will only speak of perfect health.

MY CANCER DIARY

"Words are, of course, the most powerful drugs used by mankind."

Rudyard Kipling

Date:

Appointments:

Results/Reports:

Prescriptions:

Things to do:

Thoughts:

Meditation:

Today I will use the power of my words to promote my healing.

MY CANCER DIARY

"Medical science tells us that people with a determined, feisty spirit usually get well quicker than people who are prone to be negative and discouraged...A negative spirit dries up your energy; it weakens your immune system."

Joel Osteen, pastor
author, YOUR BEST LIFE NOW

Date:

Appointments:

Results/Reports:

Prescriptions:

Things to do:

Thoughts:

Meditation:

My spirit soars. I will never be discouraged.

MY CANCER DIARY

"Life is a series of experiences, each one of which makes us bigger, even though it is hard to realize this. For the world was built to develop character."

Henry Ford

Date:

Appointments:

Results/Reports:

Prescriptions:

Things to do:

Thoughts:

Meditation:

I grow stronger in health and character each day.

MY CANCER DIARY

"Adversity often pushes us into our divine destiny. Many people respond negatively to adversities and trouble, rather than believing that God can bring good out of the situation I'm not saying God sends the trouble, but I say God will use any adversity you face to take you to a higher level if you'll just do your part and keep standing strong."

Joel Osteen, pastor
author, YOUR BEST LIFE NOW

Date:

Appointments:

Results/Reports:

Prescriptions:

Things to do:

Thoughts:

Meditation:

Today I will stand strong.

MY CANCER DIARY

"Things themselves touch not the soul, not in the least degree, nor have they admission to the soul, nor can they turn or move the soul, but the soul moves itself alone, and whatever judgments it may think proper to make, it makes for itself the things which presents themselves to it."

Marcus Aurelius, Emperor of Rome   (AD 121-180)

Date

Appointments:

Results/Reports:

Prescriptions:

Things to do:

Thoughts:

Meditation:

I will trust in the judgment of my soul. My soul is all powerful.

MY CANCER DIARY

"When we do the best that we can, we never know what miracle is wrought in our life, or in the life of another."

Helen Keller

Date:

Appointments:

Results/Reports:

Prescriptions:

Things to do:

Thoughts:

Meditation:

Today, I will do the best I can.

MY CANCER DIARY

"Obstacles cannot crush me. Every obstacle yields to my stern resolve. He who is fixed on a star does not change."

Leonardo da Vinci

Date:

Appointments:

Results/Reports:

Prescriptions:

Things to do:

Thoughts:

Meditation:

I will overcome every setback, every day.

MY CANCER DIARY

"Enlarge your vision. Develop a healthy self-image. Discover your power of thoughts and words. Stand strong against opposition and adversity. Live to give, Make a choice to be happy."

Joel Osteen, pastor
author, YOUR BEST LIFE NOW

Date:

Appointments:

Results/Reports:

Prescriptions:

Things to do:

Thoughts:

Meditation:

I choose to rise above all negative thoughts and be happy.

MY CANCER DIARY

"In some quarters, intention is synonymous with prayer, and prayer is synonymous with healing when you send out an intention"

Lynne McTaggart
author, THE INTENTION EXPERIMENT

Date:

Appointments:

Results/Reports:

Prescriptions:

Things to do:

Thoughts:

Meditation:

I intend to live a wonderful life.

MY CANCER DIARY

We are not being called upon to rearrange the planets in the sky or to alter the composition of the sun. We are called upon to make decisions affecting our own welfare. The only price we have to pay for survival is decision. "

Norman Cousins, cancer survivor
author, ANATOMY OF AN ILLNESS

Date:

Appointments:

Results/Reports:

Prescriptions:

Things to do:

Thoughts:

Meditation:

I will survive and I will flourish

MY CANCER DIARY

"Cancer is a family affair. It affects the family so profoundly that it makes us re-evaluate what we hold dearest."

Ann Jillian, actress, cancer survivor

Date:

Appointments:

Results/Reports:

Prescriptions:

Things to do:

Thoughts:

Meditation:

Today I will focus on the ones I love.

MY CANCER DIARY

"God gives us unexpected challenges sometimes, but you'll get through it all. It's alright to cry, but not for too long."

Betty Ford, cancer survivor
Wife of President Gerald Ford

Date:

Appointments:

Results/Reports:

Prescriptions:

Things to do:

Thoughts:

Meditation:

I am positive and I am strong.

MY CANCER DIARY

"My contemplation of life...had sought me that he who cannot change the very fabric of his thought...at a deeper level and perhaps subtler level than the conscious level...will never be able to change reality, and will never, therefore make any progress."

Anwar Sadat, President
Egypt from 1970-1981

Date:

Appointments:

Results/Reports:

Prescriptions:

Things to do:

Thoughts:

Meditation:

I control my thinking, and I control my life.

367

MY CANCER DIARY

"We are raised to think of miracles as unique, rate occurrences that few people deserve. Our familiarity with miracles is limited, particularly if we define them as dramatic healings, being saved from a near accident or winning a great deal of money. Now we are learning that miracles are available to all of us all the time. What do we need to make a miracle? Willingness. A change of the mind..."

Karen Casey
author, THE COURSE

Date:

Appointments:

Results/Reports:

Prescriptions:

Things to do:

Thoughts:

Meditation:

Today I will make my own miracles.

MY CANCER DIARY

"In every pain let this thought be present, that there is no dishonor in it, nor does it make governing intelligence worse, for it does not damage the intelligence...Pain is neither intolerable nor everlasting"

**Marcus Aurelius, Emperor
of Rome   (AD 121-180)**

Date:

Appointments:

Results/Reports:

Prescriptions:

Things to do:

Thoughts:

Meditation:

I will not accept pain today.

MY CANCER DIARY

"Taking charge of yourself involves more than simply trying on new thoughts for size. It requires a determination to be happy and to challenge and destroy each and every thought that creates self-immobilizing unhappiness in you."

Wayne Dyer, PhD
author, YOUR ERRONEOUS ZONES

Date:

Appointments:

Results/Reports:

Prescriptions:

Things to do:

Thoughts:

Meditation:

I will not destroy all negative thoughts today.

MY CANCER DIARY

"People are always blaming their circumstances for what they are. I don't believe in circumstances. The people who get on in this world are people who get up and look for circumstances they want, and if they can't find them, make them."

George Bernard Shaw, playwright
MRS. WARREN'S PROFESSION

Date:

Appointments:

Results/Reports:

Prescriptions:

Things to do:

Thoughts:

Meditation:

I make my own circumstances today.

MY CANCER DIARY

"It is my belief that you can't deal with the most serious things in the world unless you understand the most amusing."

Winston Churchill

Date:

Appointments:

Results/Reports:

Prescriptions:

Things to do:

Thoughts:

Meditation:

Today I will laugh all day long.

MY CANCER DIARY

"Heart patients had a 25-30 percent reduction in adverse outcomes: death, heart failure or need for repeat angioplasty. But of all the alternative therapies employed, prayer had the most profound effect."

Lynne McTaggart
author, THE INTENTION EXPERIMENT

Date:

Appointments:

Results/Reports:

Prescriptions:

Things to do:

Thoughts:

Meditation:

I believe in the power of prayer to heal me.

MY CANCER DIARY

"If we know that we are part of an open universe, and that our minds are a matrix of reality, we will live more creatively and powerfully."

Marilyn Ferguson
author, THE AQUARIAN CONSPIRACY

Date:

Appointments:

Results/Reports:

Prescriptions:

Things to do:

Thoughts:

Meditation:

I will use the power and energy of the universe to restore my health.

374

Suggested Reading and Resources I used throughout this diary, my cancer and my life.

Your Best Life Now by Joel Osteen,
    Warner Faith Publishers, ISBN 0-446-57784-7

Heroes and Heroines by Edited by Ray B. Browne
    Gale Research Inc. ISBN O-8103-4860-8

Oxford Dictionary of Quotations (3rd Edition)
    Oxford University Press

Your Erroneous Zones by Dr. Wayne Dyer
    Funk & Wagnall ISBN-0-308-10228-2

Metaphysical Meditations by Paramahansa Yogananda
    Self-Realization Fellowship ISBN-0-87612-041-9

The Essence of Zen, compiled by Maggie Pinkney
    The Five Mile Press ISBN 978-174124-762-6

Don't Sweat The Small Stuff by Richard Carlson, Ph. D.
    Hyperion Press,   ISBN 0-7868-8185-2

Ageless Body, Timeless Minds, by Deepak Chopra, M.D.
    Three Rivers Press   ISBN 0-517-88212-4

The Spontaneous Fulfillment of Desire by Deepak Chopra
    Random House ISBN 0-375-43220-5

Quantum Healing by Deepak Chopra, M.D.
    Batam Books ISBN 0-553-34869--8

The 7 Habits of Highly Effective People, by Stephen R. Covey
    A Fireside Book by Simon and Schuster ISBN 0-671-66398-4

Molecules of Emotion, by Candace B. Pert, Ph.D.
    Scribner Publishing ISBN 13 978-0-684-83187-9

Wisdom of the Ages by Wayne Dyer
    HarperCollins Books ISBN 0-06-019231-3

Simple Abundance by Sarah Ban Breathnach
    Warner Books ISBN 0-446-51913-8

Healthline Magazine, Stamford Hospital, Stamford Conn.

The Secret by Rhonda Byrne
> Atria Books/ Beyond Words Publishing I9SBN 13: 978-1-58270-170-7

Everyday Positive Thinking by Louise L. Hay
> Hay House, Inc. ISBN 13-978-1-4019-0295-7

Power Thoughts by Louisa L. Hay
> Hay House ISBN 13; 978-1-4019-0554-5

Heal Your Body by Louise L. Hay
> Hay House, Inc. ISBN 0-87418-05-08

The Power of Intention by Dr. Wayne W. Dyer
> Hay House, Inc. ISBN1-4019-0215-4

Out of Africa by Isak Dinesen,

> Random House, ISBN 0-679-60021-3

Creative Visualization by Shakti Gawain
> Bantan Books ISBN 0-553-27044-3

1001 Meditations by Mike George
> Duncan Baird Publishers ISBN 1-84483-127-2

Positive Energy by Judith Orloff, M.D.
> Harmony Books ISBN 0-609-61010-4

Power vs. Force, by David R. Hawkins, M.D., Ph.D.
> Hay House, Inc. ISBN 13; 978-1-56170-933-5

The World's Greatest Treasury of Health Secrets
> From the Editors of Bottom Line Publications ISBN 0-88723-357-0

The Intention Experiment, Lynne Taggart
> Free Press, Simon and Schuster ISBN 978-0-7432-7696-2

The End of Illness by David B. Agus, MD
> Free Press, Simon and Schuster ISBN 978-1-4516-1019-2

The Bible

"A human being is part of the whole, called by us the "universe," a part limited in time and space. This human being experiences itself, its thoughts and feelings as something separated from the rest-a kind of optical delusion of consciousness."

> Albert Einstein

www.ingramcontent.com/pod-product-compliance
Lightning Source LLC
Chambersburg PA
CBHW081411270326
41931CB00015B/3243

* 9 7 8 0 6 1 5 7 9 2 1 4 9 *